HOT
SEX
TIPS, TRICKS, AND LICKS

DEDICATION

This book is dedicated to Brandon who has made me laugh with excitement each and every day for the past eleven years. We're just getting started!

First published in the USA in 2013 by
Quiver, a member of
Quayside Publishing Group
100 Cummings Center
Suite 406-L
Beverly, MA 01915-6101
www.quiverbooks.com

17 16 15 14 13   1 2 3 4 5

ISBN: 978-1-59233-535-0

Digital edition published in 2013
eISBN: 978-1-61058-635-1

Library of Congress Cataloging-in-Publication Data
O'Reilly, Jessica.
  Hot sex tips, tricks, and licks : sizzling touch and tongue techniques for amazing orgasms / Jessica O'Reilly.
      p. cm.
  ISBN 978-1-59233-535-0
1. Sex instruction. 2. Orgasm. I. Title.
  HQ31.O697 2013
  613.9'6--dc23

                                                        2012030398

Cover design by Traffic Design Consultants Ltd.
Photography by Holly Randall Photography

Printed and bound in Singapore

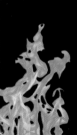

HOT SEX

TIPS, TRICKS, AND LICKS

SIZZLING TOUCH AND TONGUE TECHNIQUES
FOR AMAZING ORGASMS

JESSICA O'REILLY, Ph.D.

QUIVER

CONTENTS

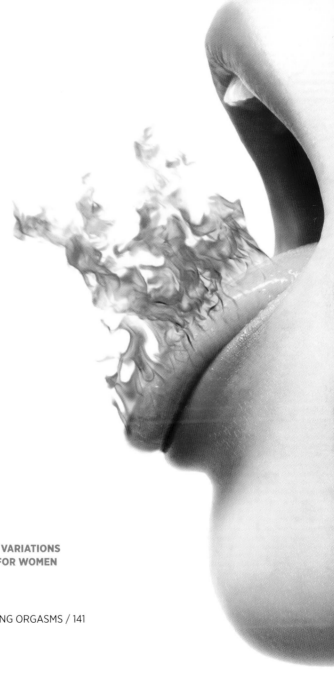

INTRODUCTION:

FINGERS AND LIPS AND TONGUES, OH MY!

DO YOU WANT TO GIVE AND GET BIGGER, BETTER ORGASMS? OF COURSE YOU DO.

You love sex—and you're already great at it—but no matter how skillful you may be there is always more to learn. That's where this book comes in. With advanced tips for skilled lovers and sexy techniques to turn your fingers, lips, and tongues into conduits of undeniable pleasure, you can enjoy the greatest sex of your life and leave your partner craving more of what you've got to give.

Mind-blowing sex isn't just about intercourse, and for many men and women the hottest and most satisfying orgasms come from tantalizing manual and oral stimulation. That's right: Your fingers, lips, and tongue are the keys to being the best lover your partner could possibly dream of. And because it's just as fun to give as it is to receive, this one-stop manual covers tips for men *and* women to make sure you're well on your way to discovering:

- The hottest erogenous zones and how to make them tingle with orgasmic pleasure
- New and innovative ways to turn your fingers into the most sought-after sex toys on the market
- Technical secrets to mind-blowing oral that may just leave plain old intercourse trailing in the dust
- Essential tips for better sex—it's not all about the technical components
- Seduction and dirty-talk techniques to get into your partner's head and fulfill his or her every desire
- Positions that pack the most power for mutual pleasure
- An appetite for exploring new fantasies and expanding your sexual horizons

These step-by-step sex tips, tricks, and licks are divided into separate sections for men and women. They're also categorized according to where they fall in the sexual response cycle: *Hot Moves to Rile Them Up* are perfect for warming up and making the body tingle with desire; *Hotter Tricks to Rock Her World* and *Drive Him Wild* are designed to bring you to the very edge of orgasm; *the Hottest Techniques for Mind-Blowing Orgasms* are sure-fire ways to make your lover moan with pleasure and dream of you and your sexual skills for years to come.

With more than a hundred techniques, variations, and tips, you can't possibly cover them all in one sitting—no matter how ambitious you are! So pick and choose from the hottest hand tricks and tongue licks and have fun experimenting with new ways to take your sexual experience and connection to new heights.

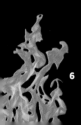

Please Read! This Is a No-Pressure Zone

This book is full of tips and techniques to thrust your sex life into high gear. But it isn't intended to be the be-all, end-all of all things sexual. Quite the opposite: Its intention is to inspire you to broaden your sexual horizons, change up your routine, and talk about your most carnal desires, fears, and fantasies.

None of these tips, tricks, and licks is designed to define your sexuality or add to the already immense pressure that exists to be "perfect" at sex. In fact, one of the most important strategies for revolutionizing your sex life is to ditch the pressure. We experience so much pressure when it comes to sex that we expend energy challenging our performance at every turn: *Am I doing it right? Does my lover like it? How do I look? Did my partner have an orgasm? Am I big enough, strong enough, hot enough, tight enough, wet enough, hard enough?* The list goes on and on and on.

But sex shouldn't be a performance; it should be an experience. You don't need to be a master of every imaginable sexual trade to knock your lover's socks off. You can be great in bed without embracing every single sex move under the sun—that's why there are so many options! Take in as much or as little as you like and change your mind as often as you want. The good news is that with every technique detailed in these pages, you just can't screw up because every move is a new discovery.

Whatever your fancy, rest assured that by delving into the folds of some healthy adult education, you're already on the right track.

10 Tips for Better Sex

Before you get started with the specific tips, tricks, and lick techniques, there are a few overarching guidelines that generally make for sizzling-hot sex. The technical components described in the upcoming chapters may *feel* great and make you look like a sexual rock star, but **it is the way you *think* about sex that really makes you a great lover**—for yourself and for your partners. While each person is unique and the only sure-fire way to know what your partner likes is to ask, these ten tips should have you well on your way to relishing the greatest sex of your life:

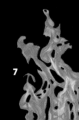

1. MAKE FOREPLAY (AKA FLIRTING) A DAILY ROUTINE.

You've probably heard about foreplay a thousand times over, but the finest foreplay isn't just about making out and some under-the-blouse groping. In fact, the hottest foreplay often doesn't involve any physical contact at all. That's right! Lusty foreplay is all about flirting with your partner in a purposeful manner intended to titillate, arouse, and eventually satisfy your mutual cravings.

Flirting is one of the most fundamental human behaviors, and each of us is hardwired to seduce prospective partners with flirtatious gestures and expressions. When you first meet, the flirting meter flies off the charts, but this sexy courting ritual wanes with time and can easily disappear even in loving relationships. This can be catastrophic, as evolutionary psychologists believe that flirting with your partner is actually a genetic survival tactic. Translation? Flirting leads to more sex!

Here are a few flirting tips to take your prolonged foreplay to new heights:

- **Touch!** Brush your hand against your lover's thigh in nonsexual situations to make the blood rush to his or her pelvic region and give your lover a taste of what's to come later. This isn't a commitment to have sex when you get home—it's just a reminder to your lover that your attraction to him or her is still red hot.

- **Be unpredictable.** Surprise your honey with sexy texts, love notes, or unannounced lunch dates. Again, sex doesn't have to be on the table for you to enjoy some intimacy, romance, and sexual tension. The power of suggestion can sometimes be as hot as sex itself.

- **Offer compliments.** This is an easy one! If you're new to flirting or feel awkward dishing out sexy talk, begin with compliments of an animalistic nature. While lustily running your eyes over your honey's body, tell your lover how much you love his or her skin, eyes, thighs, arms, or any other feature you're genuinely attracted to.

- **Whisper!** Almost anything sounds sexy when you lower your voice. So the next time you two are eating dinner together, walk over to your partner's side and whisper sweet nothings in his or her ear.

- **Dress the part.** A three-piece suit or spiky stilettos may not always be practical, but if you want to turn on the flirt, you need to *feel* sexy. So make a point of dressing up in outfits, underwear, and shoes that make you feel seductive and irresistible. And when your partner goes out of his or her way to dress to impress you, be sure to lay on the flattery to show your appreciation for the effort.

- **Be playful!** Flirting doesn't have to be serious business; in fact, it should be fun! Don't worry about saying everything perfectly, and make light of any blunders, awkward moments, or mishaps. Laughter and sex actually have a lot in common, as they both are accompanied by a surge in endorphins. And since laughter helps to break tension, it may just be the relaxant you need to enjoy an evening (or morning) of sexual intimacy.

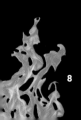

Anyone who has ever enjoyed a passionate courtship will tell you that the chase can be just as hot as the prize. So enjoy the journey for what it is.

2. GET ORAL!

Oral sex isn't always about getting on your knees and puckering up. Some of the best oral sex (think long-term payoff) can be taken care of standing up or sitting at the dinner table—through real, honest communication. Getting oral with your partner is probably *the* most important thing you can do to cultivate a red-hot sexual relationship. So start talking!

It may not be easy to do, but the more you practice the easier it gets. If a topic is awkward, use these four tips to get started:

- **Talk when the time is right.** Initiating a serious conversation about sex right before you're about to get hot and heavy isn't always an ideal. You're more likely to rush through the discussion if you're goal is really to get down to business. So set some time aside when sex is off the table: Start talking about sex while you're out for coffee, having lunch, or driving to work.
- **Be honest with yourself first.** To communicate effectively with your partner, you first need to know exactly what you want. So take some time to jot down your needs as well as your biggest fears. Bring these to the table when you talk to your partner and be honest about your vulnerabilities and uncertainties. Talking openly about your insecurities helps your partner understand your perspective and reduces the likelihood that you'll manifest those issues in an untoward (and less attractive) manner at a later date.
- **Make requests—not complaints.** Talk about your hottest turn-ons and steadfast turn-offs, but be mindful that sex is a highly sensitive subject. Frame your statements in terms of personal feelings as opposed to attacks and accusations. If there is something your partner does that drives you crazy (and not in a good way), try expressing yourself in terms of preference rather than criticism: "I prefer when you suck hard as opposed to tickling with just the tip of your tongue." Straightforwardness and tact need not be mutually exclusive.
- **Listen and ask questions.** The sex talk will be easier and smoother if it's a two-way exchange as opposed to a lecture. If you're naturally more inclined toward verbal expression than your partner, take a step back and encourage him or her to open up so the conversations isn't one-sided. Listen intently and ask for clarification as needed.

Those who report the highest levels of sexual satisfaction often spend more time *talking* about sex than *having* sex. Some even say that serious sexual conversations increase their sex drive because their erotic juices start flowing in their minds, lips, and bodies.

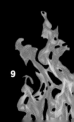

3. TALK DIRTY.

If new moves, techniques, and positions set off a flurry of sexual response in your partner's body, then a little sexy talk will launch his or her arousal into an explosive new universe. The mind really is the most powerful sex organ, and if you can tap into your partner's primal sexual mind, then you'll be the best lover he or she has ever had.

Sexy talk doesn't have to be vulgar or obscene. (Although if that's your thing, embrace it!) It can be alluring, aggressive, responsive, ego-stroking, instructive, descriptive, naughty, or fantastical. Find your comfort zone and clearly communicate your boundaries. Read through these sexy one-liners and try them on your partner—they will have your partner's head spinning with sexual satisfaction.

Alluring and Teasing
- I know you want what's under this shirt.
- Want to come play with me?
- Make me come!
- I'll do whatever you tell me to do.

Aggressive
- I'm going to hold you down and make you come.
- Can you handle what I'm about to do?

Responsive
- Tell me how you like it. I'll do whatever you tell me.
- What can I do for you?
- I'm just going to lay back and let you work me over.

Ego Stroking
- You're the best I've ever had.
- You make me so wet/horny/excited/hard.
- Tell me you want me./Tell me how sexy I am.
- You're so hot. I just want to tear through your clothes to get at that body.

Demanding and Instructive
- Give it to me how I like it.
- Tell me what you're going to do to me.
- Put your hands on my hips and bend me over. I want you to make me moan.
- Get on your knees and do it how I like it.

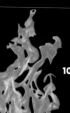

Descriptive
- I'm going to put my lips and tongue exactly where you like it.
- I'm touching myself. It feels so good.
- I'm coming!

A Little Naughty
- I want to taste you.
- I thought about you last night when I was touching myself.
- Tie me down and have your way with me.

Fantastical
- You're so good. I want to share you and watch you please another man/woman.
- I bet you'd get rock hard/soaking wet if we had a little threesome.

4. UNLEARN. FORGET EVERYTHING YOU'VE LEARNED FROM MAINSTREAM PORN.

Pornographic videos can be titillating, exciting, and entertaining. And for most of us, they're the closest thing to live sex we've ever seen, so it's natural that we pick up some tips and beliefs about sex from them. The problem with this natural "learning" is that mainstream porn is not intended to be educational. Accordingly, porn's representations of the human body, sexual response, orgasm, positions, and sexual interactions are not always accurate or typical.

Here are a few basic porn reeducation lessons that will help you look at your own sex life more realistically:

- Women don't always scream to the point of breaking glass when they have orgasms. These are porn-gasms and are not representative of most real orgasms, which often fall between the extremes of a gentle exhale and earth-shattering screams. *Note:* The latest research confirms that the sounds women make during sex often do not correspond to their orgasms and experiences of pleasure.
- Men and women both require some warming up before penetrative sex. Sex scenes involve a whole heap of preparation from fluffing and massaging to makeup and enemas, but these necessary arrangements never make it to the final cut. This leaves the false impression that we are all raring to go at the drop of a dime, when in reality foreplay is a requisite norm for penetration. Anal sex is the perfect example of porn's miseducation. You can't just start shoving things up your butt without some serious warm-up and relaxation.
- Men lose their erections. That's life, and it's perfectly okay. It will happen to every man at some point in his life. Porn stars have fluffers on the sidelines who help keep them hard, and they also have directors who allow them to cut and restart scenes and reposition off-camera.

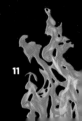

- Porn is make-believe. As adults we know the difference between fantasy and reality. Just like blockbuster movies are full of actors and special effects, so too are most X-rated films. Adult performers are sexual superstars with specialized training, resources, and experience. Trying to emulate them is a lost cause.
- You don't need to look like a porn star. And your partner probably doesn't want you to, either. With lifts, tucks, injections, bleaches, cosmetic tattoos, genetic compositions, and surgeries you've likely never heard of, most adult performers are not representative of your average—but equally sexy—man or woman.

5. GET COMFORTABLE WITH YOUR BODY.

You can't enjoy sex to its fullest potential if you're too busy worrying about how you look in a certain light or position. Focus on developing a positive body image as part of your complete lifestyle with these tips:

- Get active. Exercise is not necessarily about gaining or losing weight, but about connecting with your body in a meaningful way. It can improve circulation, elevate your mood, and make you feel better about your body. Research continues to confirm that men and women who work out feel sexier and rate themselves as better in bed.
- Eat a balanced diet. Again, this isn't about changing the way you look, but altering the way you feel. You're not likely to feel frisky after downing a triple-patty burger with fries.
- Touch yourself. Spend some time getting to know your body and learning to appreciate its unique textures, curves, and responses. If your touch becomes sexual, then roll with it; if not, just enjoy the ride.
- Build self-esteem in non-body-related arenas. Take a course, join a club, or learn a new skill to build self-confidence. And always surround yourself with people who bring out the best in you. You deserve nothing less.

DR. JESS SUGGESTS . . .

Body image is less about how you look and more about how you feel. Positive body image is also a good predictor of sexual satisfaction, so here's to loving your body and loving your orgasms!

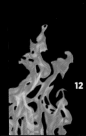

6. BE PRESENT.

Learning new techniques is a breeze compared to learning how to be present. For those of us juggling work, family, friends, and other obligations, being present during sex is no easy task. Add the pressures and distractions of technology (social media, mobile devices, GPS-tracking ankle bracelets—oh, come on, almost everyone has had to wear one at least once), and you've got a recipe for sexual disaster in which one hand is down your pants and the other is updating your status for the world to see. This may sound like a bit of an exaggeration, but recent research suggests that up to 10 percent of people actually text during sex. Really?!

Horrible texting etiquette aside, learning to be present and focus only on your current experience is a challenge even for the neo-Luddite. But with a little practice and discipline, you can learn to get your head in the game and enjoy sex to the fullest. Try out these tips for maintaining presence during steamy sex:

- Use a blindfold to heighten your sensations of touch, smell, taste, and sound while reducing visual distractions.
- Check your mobile devices at the bedroom door every day. No exceptions.
- Focus on breathing purposefully and deeply. Breath is connected to sexual response and orgasm.

DR. JESS SUGGESTS . . .

Sex researchers have found that being present is one of the key components of "optimal sex," along with communication, intimacy, and connection. Unfortunately, however, spectatoring, which involves being self-conscious and looking in at yourself from a third-person perspective, is common. It may involve judging your "performance" or worrying about your appearance instead of enjoying the sex act itself. If you catch yourself spectatoring, don't worry. Simply try to bring your thoughts back to the sexual experience by thinking about the physical sensations you're experiencing or envisioning a titillating fantasy.

- Meditate—not necessarily during sex, but on your own time to practice being present and clearing your mind.
- Slow down. Don't go straight for the genitals every time you get that primal tingle. Take time to explore the rest of the sensual body.
- Make lists. Write down all the tasks you need to complete later that day or tomorrow so you don't have dozens of thoughts and plans running through your mind when you're trying to get in the mood.
- Take it easy on yourself. You're not perfect and you never will be. There will be times when you're distracted and struggle to be present, and that's okay, too.

7. BE A VOYEUR. WATCH YOUR PARTNER ORGASM.

Do you want to learn how much pressure she likes or how fast he likes to stroke it right before orgasm? Then ask your partner to put on a little show for you or take you by the hand right before he or she is about to come. No two people are the same, and we're only experts in ourselves, so watching your lover get off is the best way to find out exactly how he or she likes it. Not only is it a great learning experience, but being a self-pleasure voyeur is also really hot and intimate.

8. BE SELFISH: ONLY DO WHAT YOU LIKE.

This should be an easy one. Sex is better when you're enthusiastic, but how do you express your enthusiasm? Simple: Be authentic. If you're in the mood to go down on your partner or climb on top for the ride of your life, then dive right in. But if you're not—don't do it. You should never feel obligated to do anything sexually. That's not to say that you shouldn't work to cultivate desire (with yourself and with your partner), but if you're not feeling it, just back off and enjoy some nonsexual snuggling, kissing, caressing, and hugging. No pressure.

9. GIVE FEEDBACK.

There is nothing worse than climbing atop what the French call *une etoile*—a partner who lies on his or her back like a star with no movement or response. Showing appreciation for your lover's efforts is just as critical to your own sexual satisfaction as asking for what you want. Tell your lover how much you love being sexual with him or her by using your words, facial expressions, sounds, and body language.

You wouldn't like to go down on your partner and wonder wheather he or she is enjoying it or nodding off into a deep sleep, would you? A soft smile, moan, prolonged exhale, or caress goes a long way toward letting your lover know how good it feels.

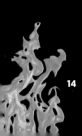

10. USE LUBE.

If you've never used lube for sex play, it will change your life! Seriously. Fingering, hand jobs, blow jobs, cunnilingus, erotic massage, anal play, and any other sex act you can dream up are taken to new heights with a little slippery lube. For most of the tips, tricks, and techniques described in this book, lube is an absolute necessity—in fact, you could easily hurt yourself without it, so take a moment to read through the section on Getting Wet and Wild (page 18).

Positions That Please

Sex feels better when you're comfortable, and finding the right position during manual and oral sex will affect how long you last and how much you like it. Certain techniques may be more comfortable and pack a greater pleasure punch in particular positions, so each of the upcoming hot tips, tricks, and licks includes a positioning recommendation. Bear in mind that you know your body the best, so experiment, be gentle, and make adjustments to accommodate your specific needs.

THE DOG

Just because this position is pretty self-explanatory doesn't mean it's a bore. Quite the opposite! The Dog allows your partner to access your hot, pulsing nether regions from both the front and the back and makes it easy for you to control the pressure and depth.

- Get down on all fours (hands and knees) and be on your best behavior to earn a ravishing treat.
- Your partner can approach from behind or lie beneath you on his or her back.

GIMME MORE

Are you more of a taker or a giver? As a lover, it is imperative to know how to play both roles and the Gimme More position encourages you to sit back, relax, and enjoy the ride.

- Sit on your bum with your back resting against the wall or headboard of your bed.
- Bend your knees and spread your legs open with your feet flat against the floor or mattress.
- Enjoy the view or ask for a blindfold to heighten your touch, smell, and sound sensations.

DIRECTOR'S CHAIR

Giving directions is about more than just spewing orders. You can easily communicate your wants, needs, and fantasies using your body language alone.

- Sit upright in a chair with your legs spread apart.
- Place a pillow at your feet and guide your kneeling partner's hands and mouth toward your sweet spots.

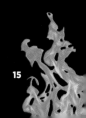

FACE DOWN, BUM UP!

Feeling lazy, but still want to get it on? Then this is the position for you. It not only combines the excitement of a rear-entry approach, but it also allows you to experience new sensations and play with the vulnerability of being pleasured from behind.

- Lie on your stomach with your hips propped up on a pillow.
- If you're a screamer and want to stay on good terms with your nosy (and jealous) neighbors, you may also want to put your face in a pillow to muffle some of your more explicit sounds.

LIE BACK AND TAKE IT

Research indicates that the ability to relax is positively correlated with both orgasm and sexual satisfaction. So a little rest and relaxation may be just what the Sex Doctor ordered. The Lie Back and Take It position forces you to take a more passive role (at least physically—you can always get active with some sultry dirty talk while you're lying there) and relish in the refined delight of being pleased.

- Lie on your back and spread your legs. Seriously. That's it!

SPREAD EAGLE

This position is a slight variation of the Lie Back and Take It.

- Simply lie on your back with your legs spread open and place a pillow under your hips to prop them up. This will allow easier access to your lower genitals, perineum, and bum hole.

SIT ON MY FACE

Not only is this position sizzling hot in terms of the view for both parties, but it's great for the sitter because he or she can control the also depth of pressure, speed, and penetration depth. If you like to play with a little dominance and submission, the Sit on My Face position is a sexy way to receive oral while maintaining a dominant role.

- Have one partner lie on his or her back and get comfortable, adding pillows to support the head, neck, and knees as needed.
- The other partner kneels over his or her partner's head, facing up toward the top of his or her head.

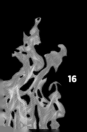

STAND AT ATTENTION

Standing up for sex not only varies your body's interpretations of sexual pleasure, but it also makes for great opportunities for sex outside of the bedroom. While a mattress may be the comfiest option, there is nothing hotter than slipping away for a secret rendezvous at a wedding, an office function, a fiftieth anniversary party, or a school concert. And since carrying an inflatable mattress is neither practical nor inconspicuous (emphasis on secret rendezvous), learning to Stand at Attention even when you're frenzied and weak in the knees may just become an essential life skill.

- Stand with your feet hip-distance apart while your partner gets on his or her knees between your legs.
- Don't let those knees buckle!

SWING SET

Your bedroom should be a playground for erotic exploration, and what playground would be complete without a Swing Set?

- Lie back, relax and let you lover do all the work as your legs swing with pleasure.
- If you're feeling particularly tender, place a pillow on the floor between your legs to protect your lover's knees.

THE LUSTY T

Some sexual techniques are just better when you approach from the side. If you're going down on a woman, it may be easier to play with the grooves of her sensitive labia; if you're going down on a man, a sideways approach can give your tongue easy access to one of the most sensitive parts of his penis: the frenulum.

- Have your partner lie on his or her back with a pillow propping up his or her hips.
- Lie on your stomach at a 90-degree angle and bury your head in his or her crotch.

REVERSE COWGIRL

If you're into real estate, then the Reverse Cowgirl has everything you could possible dream of: a great view, a convenient location with easy access, and top value for your sex-play dollar. But the best part about this position is that it maximizes pleasure for both of you, thus promoting dual orgasms. As the Cowgirl bends forward to work her magic, her lover can tease and tantalize her from behind with his fingers or her favorite toy.

- The man lies on his back while the woman straddles him over his chest, facing toward his feet.

The Reverse Cowboy is a variation in which the woman lies on her back and the man straddles her on his knees.

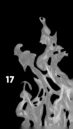

GIRAFFE

Deep-throating gets a lot of press in the world of porn and popular culture magazines, but the reality is that it is more of a novelty than a necessity. However, ladies, if you do want to swallow his cock down your throat, elongating your neck may make you more comfortable. With some practice, relaxation, confidence, and a little help from the Giraffe position, taking him deep can become a sexual pastime you both enjoy.

- The woman lies on her back with her head hanging off the side of the bed.
- The man stands on the floor in front of her while she places her hands against his thighs to control the depth of penetration.

Be sure to check out Sharing Is Caring (page 131) for ideas that allow you to experience giving and taking simultaneously.

Getting Wet and Wild

Sex is supposed to be messy! And all that sticky, delicious goodness is only enhanced by the use of a good-quality lube. If you want to twist, twirl, suck, and slide, keep lube on hand at all times. It heightens pleasure by allowing you to play with more advanced tricks and techniques that would otherwise be painful or dangerous—and it reduces friction to make sex safer.

Water-based lubes offer a consistency similar to that of vaginal lubrication but with more staying power. They wash away easily in the shower or bath, so they're not ideal for underwater sex, but they won't stain your sheets and are safe to use with condoms and sex toys. If you're prone to yeast infections, you may want to pick a glycerin-free formula.

Silicone-based lubes are super-slippery and longer lasting. With an oil-like texture (but no actual oil), they're condom compatible, great for shower play, and ideal for hand jobs. Silicone lubes should not be used with silicone sex toys. You'll also want to test to make sure they don't stain your bed sheets.

DR. JESS SUGGESTS . . .

If your water-based lube starts to dry out, just add a few drops of water to make it last longer.

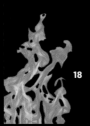

Flavored lubes are great for oral sex, and some of the organic brands are now producing more subtle flavors that actually taste good!

Whichever lube you choose, test it out on your skin first. If the sex is hot, it will likely get on your face, chest, hands, mouth, genitals, and maybe even your toes if you're lucky—so pick a brand that tastes good and contains natural ingredients.

SOME WAYS TO HAVE FUN GETTING WET AND WILD

- Rub lube on your lips and then use your wet lips to spread it all over your partner's genitals.
- Use a soft paintbrush or makeup brush to paint it all over your hot zones.
- Put some lube in the palm of your hand and make a fist, allowing the drops to trickle down your lover's thighs and pubic mound.
- Apply flavored lube in excess, and then sensually lick off some of the excess.
- Refrigerate your favorite lube for a few hours and play with the cool tingle in your mouth while you go down on your partner. Alternate with a sip of hot water or tea to play with temperature and keep your partner guessing.
- **For women:** Massage it all over your breasts as you look into your partner's eyes, and then rub your slippery boobies all over your partner's sweet spots.
- **For men:** Pour lube all over your balls and then rub them between your lover's thighs.
- Rub your hands together and use your breath to warm the lube before stroking your partner.
- Tease a little! Use lube to trace a slow line or circle around a hot spot without directly touching the erogenous zone to draw blood and awareness to the area. You can use a finger or two for this technique, or you can get more creative with your tongue, lips, nipples, or breath.
- Institute a no-hands rule for lubing up your partner.

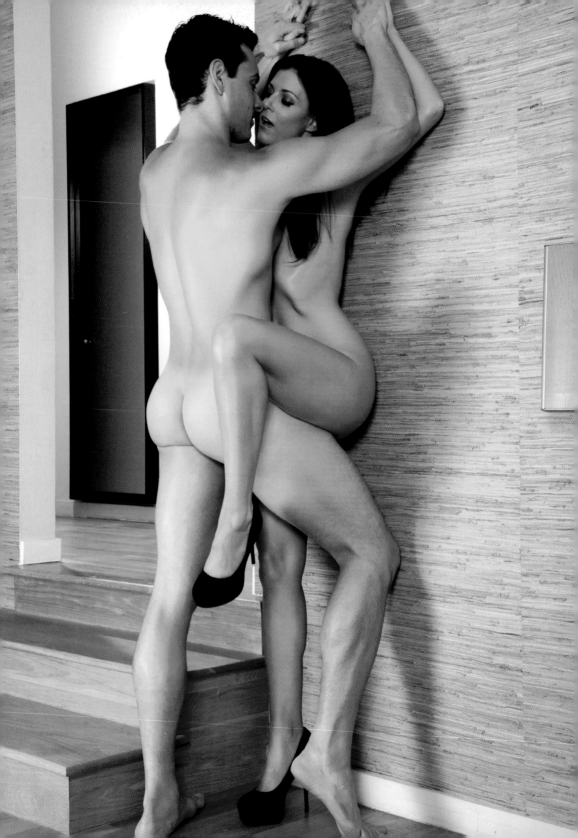

CHAPTER 1

HER SWEET SPOTS: FEMALE ANATOMY AND EROGENOUS ZONES

THE FEMALE FORM IS A BEAUTIFUL THING! And while every woman's body is unique, there are a few areas that tend to make many women purr with pleasure. As you stimulate these sensitive erogenous zones, you'll leave her skin tingling with delight and her mind wandering into exciting, unchartered territory. Pick a new one to play with each day, or set some time aside on a lazy morning to explore all of her hot spots in succession. By the time your turn comes around, she'll be aching to pay you back for those mind-blowing, full-body orgasms.

AROUND HER BODY

Her inner thighs: Maybe it's their proximity to her sweet little pussy, or perhaps it's the rich nerve endings and veins that cross paths with her genitals—whatever the case, this sweet patch of skin is often highly responsive to a gentle touch, kisses, or licks.

Her collarbone: This sexy area is a hotbed of erotic energy. Work your way outward from the collarbone and stimulate the sensitive skin under her arms.

The backs of her knees: Make her weak in the knees from the get-go by breathing gentle kisses against the skin of this oh-so-common sweet spot.

The small of her back: You may have heard of women who can reach orgasm through breast stimulation alone, but did you know that some women become aroused and orgasm from having the small of their back rubbed, licked, and passionately kissed? Use some massage oil, flavored lube, toys, or your tongue to discover how to pleasure your lady from behind, paying special attention to that sexy little indentation in the center just above her bum.

The sides of her breasts: The nipple is not the breast—but many overzealous lovers seem to hone in on this one area when in fact other parts of the breasts are just craving their sexual touch. Many women report that the sides of the breasts (near the underarm) and the area above the areola are actually the most erotic zones for kissing, licking, and sucking. Bear in mind that these twins are not actually identical—each breast differs in appearance and sexual response—so find out if she favors one over the other.

GETTING TO KNOW THE GENITALS

The vulva: This term refers to all the delicious parts on the outside of a woman's genitals.

Outer labia/lips: Protective lips containing smooth muscle, erectile tissue, fatty tissue, sweat glands, and nerve endings, the labia begin at the pubic bone at the top and come together above the perineum at the bottom, enclosing the inner labia on each side.

Inner labia/lips: Another set of lips that enclose and protect the vaginal and urethral openings, the inner labia are thin and hairless, and contain sensitive nerve endings, erectile tissue, and various glands that produce sweat, scent, and sebum (a pleasant, oily secretion).

Mons or venus mound: This soft area of fatty tissue protrudes above the pubic bone and may be covered in hair depending on grooming preferences. Touching or gently tugging on the mons can lead to some of the most overpowering orgasms, because the base of the clitoris's suspensory ligament is hidden in this very sexy mound.

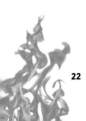

Vulva

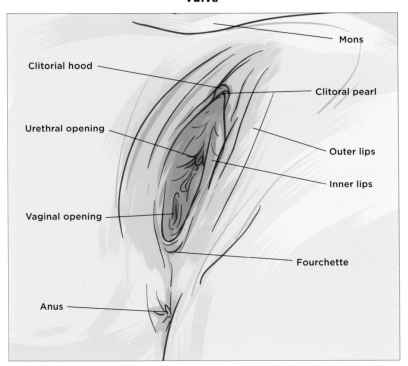

Mons

Clitorial hood

Clitoral pearl

Urethral opening

Outer lips

Inner lips

Vaginal opening

Fourchette

Anus

Clitoris: The only body part designed for the sole purpose of pleasure, the clitoris is composed of many parts, including the head, hood, shaft, legs, and bulbs. Some scientists believe that the erectile tissue in the labia and vagina (including the G-spot) are also a part of the clitoral structure.

Clitoral head or pearl: Sometimes referred to as *the* clitoris, the clitoral head is only one piece of this wondrous pleasure powerhouse. Located at the top of where the inner labia meet, the head may be hidden beneath the hood or protrude on its own.

Clitoral hood: This foreskin covers and protects the clitoral head.

Clitoral shaft: Attached to the clitoral head, this segment of erectile tissue expands downward, and when erect it wraps around the vagina on the inside of the body.

Clitoral legs: These internal legs can extend up to 3½ inches (9 cm) and point backward when erect.

Clitoral bulbs: Located beneath the outer labia, these internal bulbs fill with blood and can push the vulva outward when a woman is sexually excited.

Fourchette: This is the sensitive spot where the inner labia meet at their southernmost point.

Urethral sponge (G-spot): This is more of an area than a particular spot. Located on the upper (front) wall of the vagina, it may be hard to find when a woman is not aroused, but as she becomes excited, the area gets harder and more ridgelike as it fills with blood.

Vagina: This tubelike canal is composed of mucous membranes and enclosed by elastic tissue and muscles.

Urethral opening: This is the hole through which pee and ejaculate are expelled.

Anus: Also known as the bum hole, the anus consists of two sphincter muscles and lots of sensitive nerve endings.

Bartholin's glands: These are two small secretion glands near the bottom of the vulva, with ducts on either side of the vaginal opening. They are located under the skin and they produce a small amount of fluid to lubricate the vulva.

Perineum: This is the smooth space between the lower vulva and the anus.

ALL ABOUT HER ORGASM

The female sexual response cycle is unique and varied. Not only is each woman different, but also each experience will differ even for the same woman. The following four-part breakdown is simply a generalized guide to describe some of the physical sensations that *may* be experienced during sex play. Each of these stages and manifestations can occur independently, and sex can be just as thrilling without reaching every stage and experiencing every sensation.

DESIRE AND AROUSAL

- Thoughts turn to sex, intimacy, romance, eroticism, or physical connection—often in response to sexual stimuli.
- Heart rate and blood pressure increase.
- Labia, nipples, and clitoris fill will blood and become enlarged.
- Muscles tense up.
- Vagina lubricates.

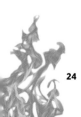

INTENSE AROUSAL

- Sex flush (red, rashlike splotches on the body) appear.
- Breathing and heart rate increase.
- The body perspires.
- Labia continue to swell and darken.
- Breasts swell, increasing in size.
- Pelvic floor muscles contract, causing tightness around the vaginal opening.
- The clitoris becomes increasingly sensitive, and the head retracts under the hood.

ORGASM

- Muscles spasm or tense up involuntarily.
- Blood pressure, breathing, and heart rate increase.
- Toes curl.
- The PC muscle and uterus contract.
- The anal sphincter contracts.
- Fluid may ejaculate from the urethra.
- Moans, screams, or deep exhalations may emanate from her lips.
- Sexual tension is released.

POSTORGASM

- Her clitoris may be hypersensitive.
- Heart rate, blood pressure, and breathing slow to nonarousal levels.
- Swollen areas (e.g., labia, clitoris, nipples, breasts, vaginal walls) return to their previous size.
- Some women like to rest and enjoy the refractory period while others will jump right back into experiences of arousal.

Note: There are many types of arousal, but the two we tend to focus on in terms of sex are *physical* and *mental* arousal. These often work hand in hand, but sometimes they operate on totally different wavelengths. This is why physical techniques are only a piece of the puzzle. To enjoy mind-blowing sex and relish the physical changes associated with sexual response, you have to get your head in the game. This is where seduction, intimacy, dirty talk, fantasy, and deepened connections come into the equation.

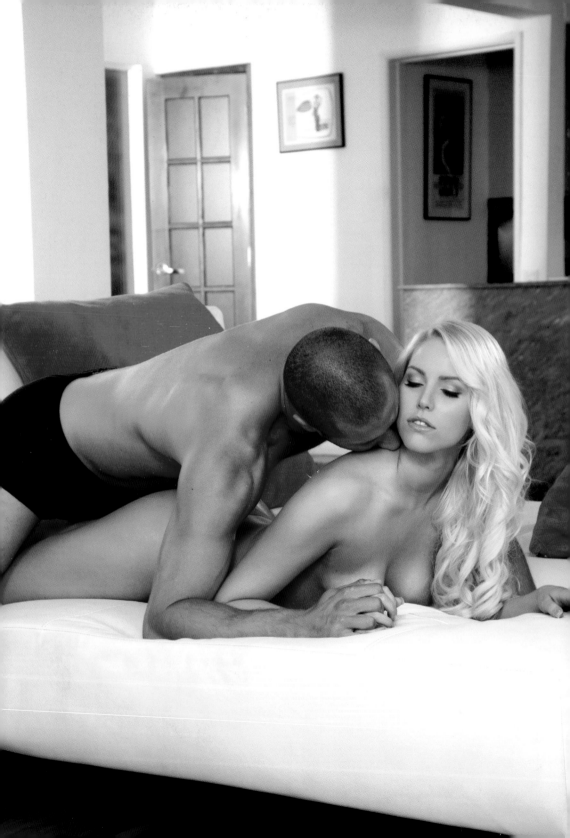

CHAPTER 2

HOT MOVES TO RILE HER UP

THESE WARM-UP MOVES will put your lady in a frisky mood and leave her begging for more. For the most part, they're not designed to bring her over the edge but rather to build up her excitement for a full-body orgasm she won't soon forget!

Practice these touches on the back of your hand or wrist ahead of time to see what feels natural for you. As you experiment, you'll find ways to adapt them to your own needs and switch them up in accordance with your woman's response.

You won't want to use them all at once—even sexual superheroes need to come up for air! And though you may be tempted to proceed at full speed toward her sure-fire hot buttons, remember that sometimes good things come to those who wait. And when it comes to sex, smaller, gentler movements can lead to big, powerful results.

PUSSY POCKET ▶

This simple move can be used to warm her up, help her relax, multiply her climactic contractions, and even calm her down postorgasm. It's a simple one, but totally indispensable.

POSITIONING

Sit next to her on the couch or straddle her in the Reverse Cowboy for easy access to her pussy.

DR. JESS SUGGESTS . . .

Try the Pussy Pocket over her clothes while you're curled up on the couch or out for dinner.

TECHNIQUE

- Place your palm on her Venus mound and cup your fingers down over her labia.
- Use your Pussy Pocket to create a wave of erotic energy by curving your fingers in a smooth, undulating motion over her vulva.
- Alternate between waves, pulses, and no movement according to her response and hip movements.

NO-HANDS MASSAGE

As hard as it may be to keep your hands off of her beautiful body, sometimes a hands-off approach is exactly what you both need to get the sparks flying.

POSITIONING

Anything goes for this one! Since your hands won't be all over her for once, you can use them to support yourself over her body. Try it with your lover in the Lie Back and Take It or Gimme More position.

TECHNIQUE

- Kiss her neck and collarbone as you blindfold her so that she can focus on the physical sensations of your touch.
- Caress her hands with any part of your body you'd like. You can use your chin, lips, ears, feet, thighs, tongue, cheek, thighs, scrotum, or even penis.

- Work your way all around her body using anything but your hands to get her all riled up. Don't forget about the backs of her knees, inner thighs, earlobes, lips, hips, and neck.

VARIATIONS AND ADVANCED TECHNIQUES

- Focus on your own pleasure, too! If you like to feel her hands against your shaft (and you probably do!), put your lubed penis right in the palm of her hand and rub yourself off a little.
- If you have a bit of facial hair, apply some oil and gently tickle her neck, chest, and ears with your sexy stubble.

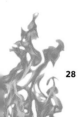

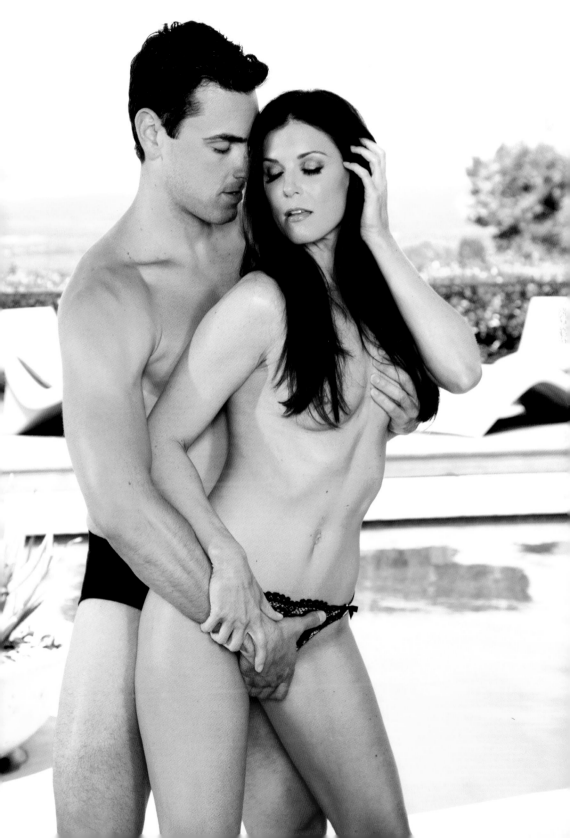

TAKE MY BREATH AWAY

Want to get her all hot and primed for an orgasm that tingles all over? Then take a page out of the ancient sex text the Kama Sutra and blow oh-so-gentle kisses her way until she's begging for more. It may be hard to resist putting your wet puckered lips against her glistening skin, but a little bit of teasing can go a long way—and will be well worth it in the end.

POSITIONING

Ask her to lie on her stomach in the Face Down, Bum Up! position so that you're able to get between her thighs.

TECHNIQUE

- Get your lips nice and wet so that she can feel the warm moisture approaching her skin.
- Start by blowing gentle kisses all over her left outer foot and ankle, bringing your lips as close to her skin as possible without making contact.
- Be sure to let out a gentle breath as you kiss so that she can feel your warmth and desire.
- Move *as slowly as possible* and continue breathing air kisses against her skin as you work your way up the outer side of her left calf, knee, and thigh.
- When you reach her hip, work your way back down the center of her left thigh, knee, calf, and ankle, paying extra attention to the heel of her foot.
- Once you reach her foot, work your way back up continuing to offer gentle breath kisses along her inner leg until you reach her vulva. Breathe a few gentle kisses over her wet lips and then repeat this pattern of breath kisses on her right leg.
- By the time you reach her vulva again, she should be relaxed, excited, and ready for more!

Note: Don't ever blow air *into* the vagina, as this could cause serious harm.

VARIATIONS AND ADVANCED TECHNIQUES

- The key to this technique is to move slowly. If you happen to have a lazy Sunday morning available, see if you can spend a full ten minutes playing with breath kisses on each leg before you dive in between her legs.
- Before beginning your breath kisses routine, use a flat open palm (no fingers) to apply her favorite scented oil or lotion to her legs. This can make her skin even more sensitive and receptive to your breath.
- Sip a hot peppermint tea before beginning your breath kisses, and she'll enjoy the tingle even more!
- If she seems to like this technique, try giving her a few suggestive breath kisses when you're out at dinner or attending a social function where sex is off the table. It should make for a good warm-up for later that night when you finally find some alone time.

VARIATION: A LOT OF HOT AIR

- If you're short on time, begin your sex session by breathing some warm air all over her thighs, labia, and clitoris. Come as close as you can and allow some brief incidental contact between her labia and your lips or nose, but tease her a little before you dive in for the goods.

DR. JESS SUGGESTS . . .

Reflexologists report that stimulating the outer foot below the anklebone increases the libido; it is a reflex area connected to the woman's ovaries and the man's testes.

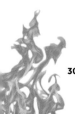

THE TONGUE TRAIL

Everyone loves a sensual back rub, and a little rubdown is a great way to help your partner wind down from a hectic day. But to make sure your massage doesn't relax her into a deep sleep, the Tongue Trail blends relaxation with titillation to help you both enjoy the best of both worlds.

POSITIONING

Ask your partner to lie in the Face Down, Bum Up! position. If you have some extra pillows, build them up around her head so that she can lie face down with some space to breathe. Straddle her at the hips and use a few pillows beneath your knees to ensure your own comfort.

TECHNIQUE

- Begin by warming up your hands with some edible massage oil or lube and gently stroking the backs of her shoulders and shoulder blades. Remember that this massage is intended to be a caress, not a therapeutic massage, so don't focus on getting deep into the muscle tissue or working out any knots.
- Use flat palms in large sweeping motions across her back and trickle your fingers gently across her underarms and sides of her chest to tease her breasts as you work your way down to her lower back.
- Breathe some warm air over the small of her back and kiss it gently with your lips.
- Draw a slow winding line (like a snake) down toward the top of her buttocks with your tongue.
- Add some lube to your mouth and slide your tongue between her bum cheeks. Work your tongue up and down the groove between her cheeks, gradually increasing the speed of your tongue strokes.
- As you slide your tongue between her bum cheeks, use your hands to squeeze them together and be sure to tell her how good it feels. If you can't seem to get your words out while you're tongue-tied between her cheeks, communicate your pleasure with some deep exhalations and moans.

VARIATIONS AND ADVANCED TECHNIQUES

Lots of people have hang-ups about their butts being touched, fingered, and kissed, so you'll need to talk to her about her comfort level. If she's comfortable with a bit of anal play (the only way to know for sure is to ask), slide your tongue all the way down to her anus and twirl it around the opening. She may be more comfortable enjoying the Tongue Trail if she has just stepped out of the shower or bath. You may even want to join her in the shower and enjoy soaping up her wet body before pressing her up against the wall and trying the Tongue Trail while standing beneath the cascading water.

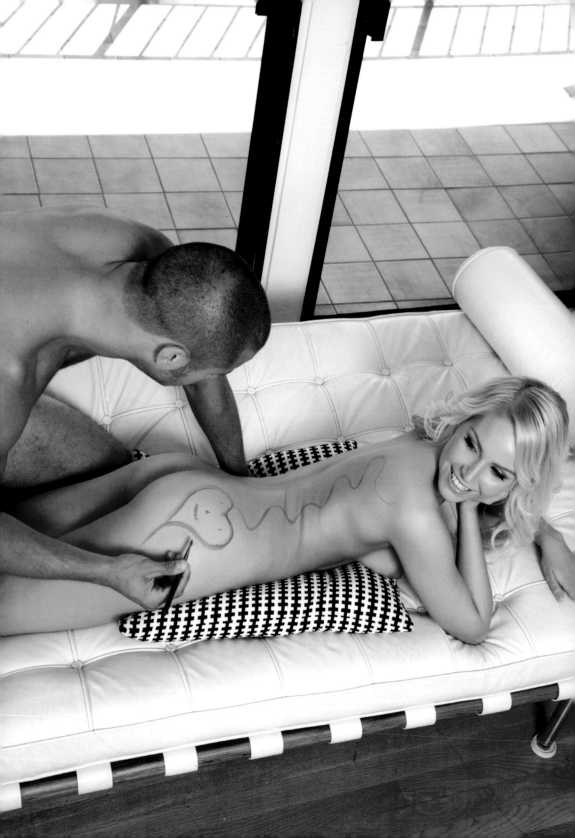

PICASSO

Whether you're a modern-day Monet or barely passed fingerpainting class back in kindergarten, the Picasso is easy to execute and totally worth the quick trip to the beauty supply store.

POSITIONING

Begin with your partner lying on her stomach in the Face Down, Bum Up! position. Tell her how much you love her body and promise her that you're going to take good care of her tonight (or this morning or afternoon).

TECHNIQUE

- Prepare for the Picasso by purchasing a soft-bristle makeup brush (about ½ inch, or 1.3 cm, thick) and some warming lube or oil.
- Dip the brush into the oil and "paint" her body, taking time to slowly approach her most sensitive parts.
- Try drawing slow, sensuous circles around her outer breasts, gradually working your way in toward her nipples. Take your time and tease her a little to leave her nipples wanting more.
- Work your way down to her vulva and paint sensuous lines between her labia and around her clitoral head and hood.
- As she becomes more aroused, stroke downward over her clitoral hood with firmer pressure to stimulate her clitoral shaft.

VARIATIONS AND ADVANCED TECHNIQUES

- Exhale some deep breaths over your "wet paint" areas.
- Try using chocolate sauce, honey, syrup, ice cream, or any other tasty treat you'd like to lick off when you're done.
- Purchase melting body candles at your local sex store and paint the hot wax over her body. Just be sure to test out the temperature on your inner wrist before getting started.
- If you're new to anal play, the Picasso may be a great way to safely explore the area around the bum hole without penetration.

DR. JESS SUGGESTS . . .

If you're hesitant to bring artistic expression into the bedroom, consider the fact that artists and those who indulge in creativity have greater sexual success and twice as many sexual partners as those who forgo creative activities.

FINGER LICK

While fingering the vagina in a traditional in-and-out motion can sometimes do the trick, most women experience fervid sexual pleasure from sexual contact with the vulva (the yummy stuff on the outside). So try to resist the urge to slide those slippery digits inside of her and go to work on her outer parts first. You may be surprised at her reaction!

POSITIONING

Sweep her off her feet and have her relax in the Gimme More position as you kneel or lie between her legs.

TECHNIQUE

- Blindfold your partner.
- Warm up your hands and get your fingers soaking wet with lube.
- "Lick" all around her wet thighs, venus mound, and outer labia with your warm, wet fingers.
- Stroke her inner labia gently in an up-and-down motion with your wet fingers so that it feels like she's being licked by several tongues.
- Use a flat wet palm to stroke up and down over her vulva as you let out a heavy breath over her clitoral head.

VARIATIONS AND ADVANCED TECHNIQUES

- Add your tongue in to the mix and play around with lube so that she can't tell the difference between your fingers and your tongue.
- Tease her and ask her if she'd like to have two or three (or more!) tongues licking her juicy pussy at the same time. If she seems to like this suggestion, tease her with fantasy talk and tell her to relax and imagine that you're sharing her pussy with someone else.
- Use two wet index fingers to stroke in opposite directions (up and down) against the sensitive skin between the inner and outer labia.

DR. JESS SUGGESTS . . .

You've probably heard that most women orgasm through clitoral stimulation, but it's not just the little head/pearl of the clitoris that's supersensitive. The bulbs and legs of the clitoris can be stimulated through the labia, so don't discount the pleasure potential of these highly responsive, liplike structures.

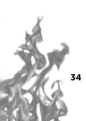

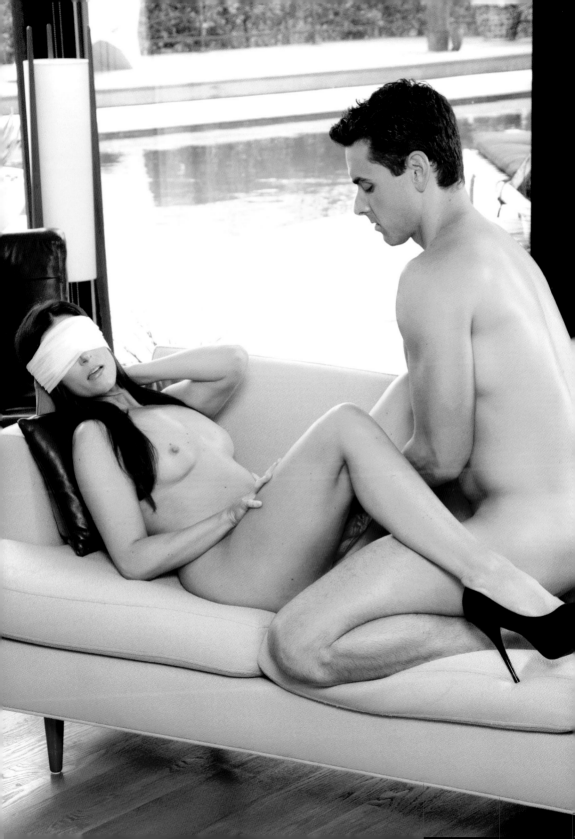

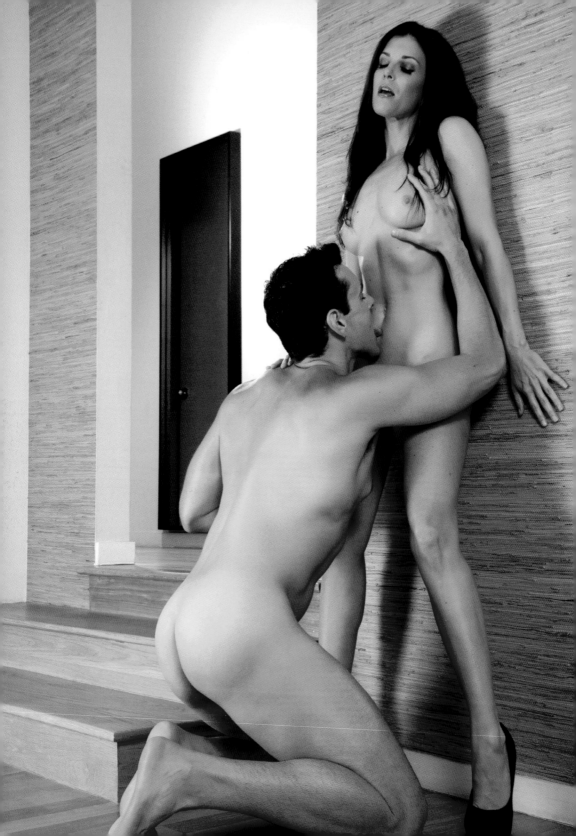

LIP LINER

This technique not only draws awareness and blood flow to the genital region, but it also traces a continuous erotic connection from the belly button all the way to the bum. By stimulating this larger area during the earlier stages of arousal, you increase the likelihood that she'll feel orgasmic sensations in this expanded zone with she comes.

POSITIONING

Try this technique with your partner in the Stand at Attention position while you kneel between her sultry thighs.

TECHNIQUE

- Circle your tongue around her belly button and tell her you love the taste as you eat it out slowly and sensually.
- Draw a line with your wet tongue (add some lube because your saliva may dry out) from her belly button to her bum hole, passing over the venus mound, clitoral hood, vaginal opening, and perineum.
- Don't spend extra time on any particular spot as you retrace your line from the anus back up to the belly button.
- Tell her how much you love the way she feels, tastes, and smells.

VARIATIONS AND ADVANCED TECHNIQUES

- Alternatively, you can use two hands (or one hand and one tongue), beginning with one at the belly button and the other at the anus. Draw each hand toward the center of the vulva simultaneously so that they meet right at the clitoral head.
- Once you've left a wet line connecting her belly button to her bum, breathe gently over the line to create a tingly sensation.

DR. JESS SUGGESTS . . .

Some women report that touching their belly button gives them pleasurable sensations in their clitoris, so the Lip Liner is a great technique to use to explore this connection.

THE POUTER

No one likes a pouter, but if you happen to be a superstar muff diver, she may be willing to overlook your sore attitude. This simple warm-up move offers a change from the traditional licking, sucking, and fingering sensations by encouraging you to use your inner lip to vary the experience.

POSITIONING

Ask her to sit in the Gimme More position and lie on your stomach between her legs.

TECHNIQUE

- Push out your bottom lip like you're a spoiled, pouty child. We know—it's a long shot, but just pretend!
- Add some lube and use that pouty lip to lick all around her inner thighs in circular motions.
- Work your way to the middle of her vulva and stroke up and down with your pout while you caress the backs of her knees with your hands.
- Try sucking on her labia while your bottom lip is still pushed out toward your chin.

VARIATIONS AND ADVANCED TECHNIQUES

While pouting with your bottom lip, poke your tongue out and upward against your upper lip so that you look like a monkey. If the monkey face makes you feel silly, just dim the lights and trust that her eyes won't be on you because they'll be rolling back into her head with pleasure. Smother her vulva with your monkey lips and moan away, resisting the urge to blurt out, "Ooh ooh, eee eee!" You can also use the monkey-face lips to suck on her nipples and nibble at her ears.

DR. JESS SUGGESTS . . .

As hot as the Pouter may be for her, it will also excite your senses, because your lips are one of your most sensitive erogenous zones. Interpreting sensations through the mental nerve, kissing your lower lip can excite a torrent of erotic energy as your blood vessels dilate, your breath and your heart rate quicken, skin flushes, and your hormone levels spike.

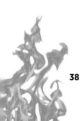

MY HEART

Vulva massage can promote circulation, encourage lubrication, and improve sexual response. But who cares about the health benefits when it feels so darn good?

POSITIONING

Ask your lady to lie on her back with her legs spread and hanging off the bed in the Swing Set position. Place a pillow on the ground between her legs and kneel between them.

TECHNIQUE

- Begin by lubing up your thumbs and placing them near the top of her venus mound.
- Use your thumbs to draw a slow heart over her mound while you insert your tongue just inside her vagina and twirl it around against the inner walls.
- Keep tongue-screwing her vagina while you draw more hearts with your thumbs, allowing them to meet at her clitoral hood and give it a very gently squeeze.
- If your tongue needs a rest, replace it with a lubed finger or two, and use the thumb of your other hand to gently encircle the clitoral head.

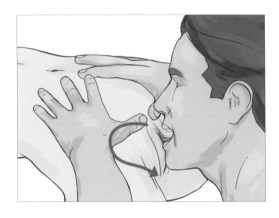

VARIATIONS AND ADVANCED TECHNIQUES

Flip her onto her stomach and tongue-screw her while you use your thumbs to draw a heart on her perineum or around her butt hole.

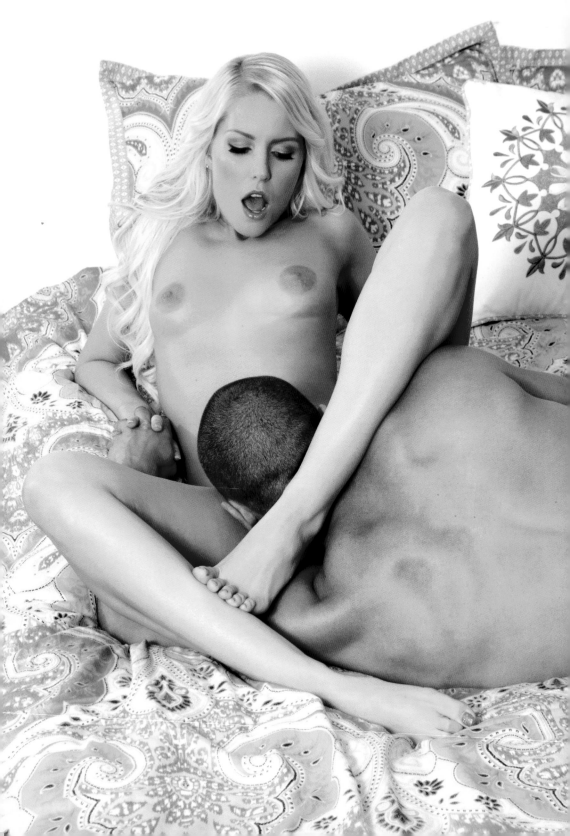

THE SUCKER

You've probably heard that pretending to lick or suck a lollipop is a great way to experiment with oral sex. But where should you begin? Try this simple move that will leave her dreaming of anything but lollipops and gumdrops.

POSITIONING

Assume the Lusty T position and, if she's flexible, have her throw one leg (the one that's closer to you) over your back so that you have greater access to her juicy goods.

TECHNIQUE

- This one is so easy if you approach from the side! Simply lick your lips and gently suck on her inner labia by pinching them together with your mouth.
- Continue sucking as you work your way from the bottom of where her labia meet up to her clitoral head.
- Close your lips into a small circle to suck on her clitoral head and hood.

VARIATIONS AND ADVANCED TECHNIQUES

If you're a great multitasker, use one hand to gently caress her underarms and the side of her breasts while the other strokes her perineum.

DR. JESS SUGGESTS . . .

The nerve endings of the vulva respond with love to subtle touch, so begin by sucking as slowly and gently as possible to get her juices flowing. Increase your suction gradually and remember to breathe and let your sounds flow naturally! Holding your breath will make you both feel tense, whereas breathing deeply promotes relaxation, connection, and pleasure.

THE VEE-JAY-JAY

This simple warm-up move will get her juices flowing and increase blood flow to her hot spots. Since you'll be stimulating her clitoris as you stroke, don't be surprised if your sexy warm-up quickly turns into some full-fledged hip thrusting and deep moaning on her part.

POSITIONING

The Vee-Jay-Jay technique is very versatile and can be performed from almost any position. For the traditional move, ask her to lie on her back with her knees bent, feet flat on the bed, and hips propped up with a few pillows. Position yourself between her legs facing up toward her beautiful vulva. She could also be seated on a chair or on the edge of the bed with her legs dangling off the side, and you can kneel on a pillow between her open legs.

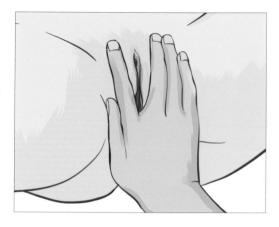

TECHNIQUE

- Apply a generous amount of lube to one hand. Remember, the wetter the better for hands-on sex!
- Lying on your stomach or kneeling between her open legs, place your wet flat palm against her vulva and spread your middle and index finger apart to form a V. Start with the vertex (bottom) of the V on the clitoral hood.
- Slide your wet palm down over her vulva to the very bottom while gently closing your index and middle fingers over her inner lips.
- Slide back up over her vulva and reopen your index and middle fingers as you approach the clitoral head and hood.
- This should become one sensual, fluid motion. Practice on your hand until it feels natural.
- Since you'll be rubbing the head, hood, bulbs, and legs of the clitoris, she'll likely press against your hand to indicate how much pressure she wants, so just follow her lead and adjust accordingly.

VARIATIONS AND ADVANCED TECHNIQUES

- Switch directions! Straddle her stomach facing her feet; start with the open V at the bottom of the vulva and work your way up to invert the sensations.
- If she is positioned on all fours, you can reach between her legs and try the Vee-Jay-Jay from behind while taking in the sexy view.
- As you close your fingers, use your lips and tongue to lick or suck on her inner lips.
- Use two hands (two Vs) to work in one direction, alternating one after the other.

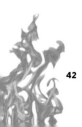

THE SENSUAL W

The Sensual W is a variation of the Vee-Jay-Jay that allows for more contact between your hands and her hot pussy.

POSITIONING

Try the Sensual W with your lover in the Swing Set position as you kneel between her legs. Change it up and take this move on the road and you'll discover unknown sweet spots and sensations with every new position.

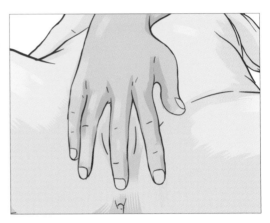

TECHNIQUE

- Place your wet palm against her vulva, but this time form a W with all five fingers (keeping your thumb together with your index finger and your pinky together with your ring finger).
- Start with your hand at the very top of her vulva and slowly slide it down toward the bottom as your squeeze your fingers together. Your middle finger can press down against her clitoris while the outer edges of the W gently squeeze her inner labia.
- Slide back up over her vulva and reopen your fingers to reform the W as you approach the clitoral head and hood.

VARIATIONS AND ADVANCED TECHNIQUES

Try the Sensual W upside down! You can alternate between a "W" and an "M" by approaching from the side in the Lusty T position or switching hands.

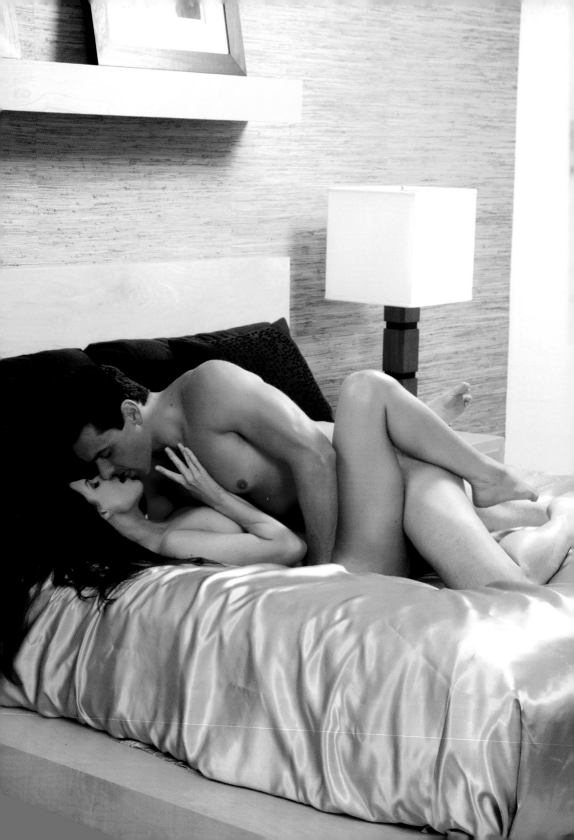

CHAPTER 3

HOTTER TRICKS TO ROCK HER WORLD

SOMEWHERE BETWEEN IRRESISTIBLE SEDUCTION and unforgettable climax lies that perfect space where she's relishing in every moment and hoping it never ends. If that's where you want to take her (for now), then these Hotter Tricks to Rock Her World are just what you're looking for. Get creative, express your primal lust, and carry her away to a point where she'll just *have to* kiss and tell.

Not only are these hotter tricks the perfect way to build toward an unforgettable climax, but they're also perfect for those nights (and mornings, and afternoons) when you don't have enough time for full-on seduction. Consider them quickie foreplay techniques that will put her in the mood and prime her for orgasm in no time at all.

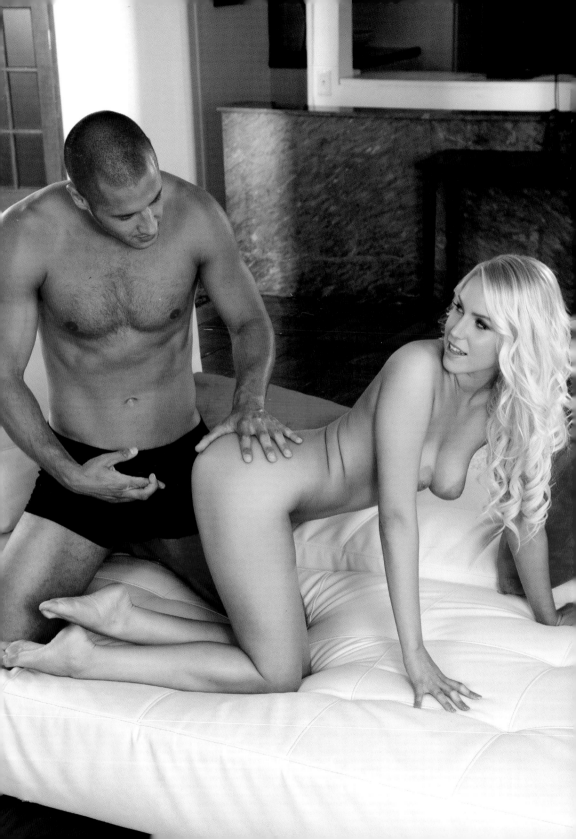

CROSS MY FINGERS

Are you dying to get inside of her and feel her warm folds surround your fingers? Of course you are! Try the Cross My Fingers technique to change things up and explore new ways to satisfy her with your bare hands.

POSITIONING

Ask her to get down on her hands and knees in the Dog position so that you get a great view from behind.

TECHNIQUE

- Begin by rubbing her bum and telling her how perfectly round, juicy, and tasty it looks from behind. Mmm!
- Cross the index and middle fingers of your dominant hand and apply some lube.
- Insert your crossed fingers into her vagina with your palm facing down.
- Once you've inserted all the way up to your second or third knuckle, rotate your hand clockwise until your palm is facing up and then pull out.
- Start slowly and increase the speed as she gets worked up—and keep telling her how much you love the view!

VARIATIONS AND ADVANCED TECHNIQUES

- As you rotate your crossed fingers, perform a scooping motion to massage the upper, lower, and sides of the vaginal walls.
- To change up the sensations, alternate your hand position to start with your palm facing upward and rotate counterclockwise as you pull out.
- Got a spare hand? Use it to play as you please. Stroke your own penis, reach around and fondle her breasts, or lick your fingers and play with the sensitive skin surrounding her bum hole.

THE ARTIST

Sex is definitely more of an art than a science, and it's a great way to express yourself. The Artist allows you to explore her sweet spots while playing with her expressive side.

POSITIONING

Ask your partner to lie Face Down, Bum Up! while you sit or lie between her legs.

TECHNIQUE

- Stroke her sides lightly with the backs of your fingers while you kiss the small of her back.
- Draw a trail of kisses down over her buttocks and use your tongue to "paint" abstract art over her bum, perineum, and vulva. Paint lines, circles, curves, swirls, angles, flowers, and any other design with a wide, flat tongue.
- Vary your "paintbrush" by tightening your tongue into a sharper point. If you want to erase your work and start again, simply use your lips to gently suck it away!

VARIATIONS AND ADVANCED TECHNIQUES

- Use a soft tongue and some tasty lube to draw flower petals all around her bum hole.
- Use a few lubed fingers at the same time as your tongue to make it feel as though she's at the center of a group-sex escapade.

DR. JESS SUGGESTS . . .

You may have heard that anal play and penetration can lead to loss of control over your bowel movements or sphincter, but this is not true for healthy adults who use lube and lots of communication. In fact, one theory suggests that those who enjoy anal penetration learn to exercise greater control over their anal muscles, resulting in greater bowel-movement control.

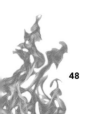

GROOVIN'

This sexy technique engages your hands and mouth to stimulate a whole series of erogenous zones between her legs, including highly responsive erectile tissue, the bulbs of the clitoris, and the sensitive glands on the inner sides of her outer lips. Yum!

POSITIONING

Prop her hips up in the Lie Back and Take It position, and lie down between her luscious legs.

TECHNIQUE

- Start with your tongue at the top of where her inner labia meet and place your thumbs at the base of her vulva.
- Use the underside of your wide, flat tongue to lick downward between her inner labia while you stroke upward with your thumbs against her outer labia.
- Vary your speed and pressure according to her arousal cues.

VARIATIONS AND ADVANCED TECHNIQUES

- Vary your thumb strokes against her outer lips to caress not only the fatty outer side, but also the gland-rich inner side of her labia majora.
- Use your nose and a bit of lube to stroke her clitoral pearl as you lick upward with your tongue.

DR. JESS SUGGESTS . . .

Learning new techniques is a great way to improve your sex life, but sex feels best when you're able to relax and focus on the sensations. Nobody wants to think about technique while they're getting it on! Because this move takes a bit of coordination, practice it ahead of time so it comes naturally and just do what feels good for you, knowing that she'll have no clue if your coordination is a bit off.

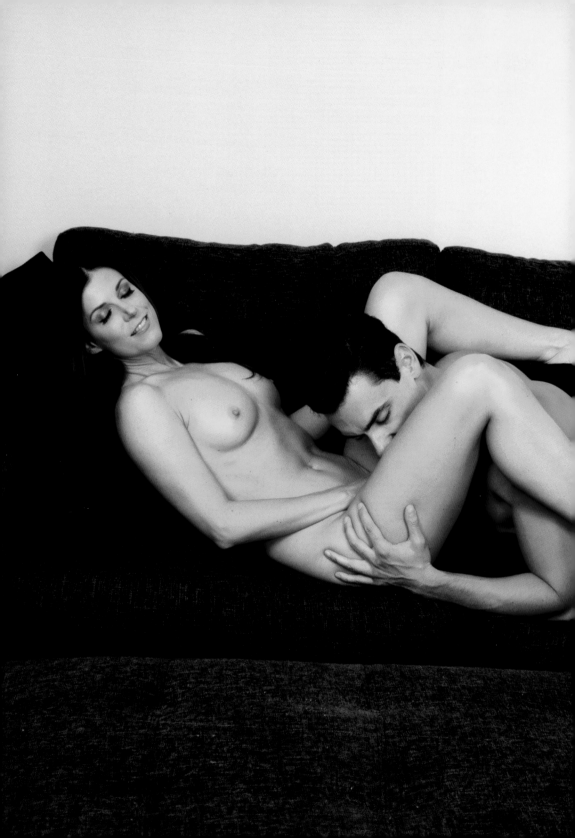

THE MULTITASKER

When you catch a glimpse of her hot body, don't you just want to ravage her? Tell her how badly you want her, and then use every part of your body (and mind) to touch, tease, tickle, suck, lick, kiss, and fondle her all over. The Multitasker is an open-ended move that encourages you to use as many parts of your body as possible at once with the goal of mutual pleasure.

POSITIONING

Try this one in the hallway of your home right when you walk in the door. You can press her up against the wall, carry her to the sofa, or lift her onto the kitchen counter.

TECHNIQUE

- Build up her anticipation during the day by sending her a few flirty text messages or emails to let her know that she's on your mind. "Thinking of you!" or "You looked hot this morning!" or "I can't wait to see you!" are a few easy examples. If you're a little more brazen in the dirty-talk department, try "I can't wait to get home and tear those panties off!" or "I thought about you wearing that black nightie and got hard under my desk this afternoon."

- On your way home, start thinking about a hot fantasy to help put you in the mood.

- When you get home, greet her with a long, deep kiss, and tell her how much you've been longing for her all day. Start undressing her and toss her clothes all over the floor.

- Pick her up and put her on the counter, couch, chair, stairs, or table. If any of these surfaces is a bit cool to the touch, plan ahead by having a throw or blanket on hand to spread beneath her.

- Once you're both in a comfortable position, go down between her legs and lick away, using one hand to play with her perineum and thighs while the other hand fondles her breasts. Try to engage as many body parts as possible.

- Take her hand and encourage her to touch herself wherever she likes (her clitoris, her bum, her breasts, her thighs).

- As you eat, suck, and fondle away, rub yourself against her legs to stroke your penis. If she likes to suck you off, flip over into the 69 position to get in on that action.

VARIATIONS AND ADVANCED TECHNIQUES

- Buy a new piece of lingerie and leave it wrapped with a bow to greet her when she gets home.

- Better yet, if she's a shoe fanatic, buy her a pair of heels and ask her to try them on for you when you get home.

- Encourage her to wrap her legs around you while you're eating her pussy so that she can thrust against you to control the speed and pressure.

DR. JESS SUGGESTS . . .

Be sure to kiss her on the lips before you leave in the morning. This will not only set the mood for a playful evening, but also research suggests that men who kiss their lovers goodbye live longer and have higher incomes. And even if this relationship isn't causal, the hormones released during a kiss can reduce stress, so you really have nothing to lose.

THUMB LOVE

Thumb Love is a hot technique that stimulates the most responsive part of her vagina—the outer third. This nerve-rich area, coined the *orgasmic platform* by early sex researchers William Masters and Virginia Johnson, swells during arousal and contracts during orgasm. Because this hot spot is located just inside the entrance of the vagina, it's also a realistic reminder that when it comes to penises, fingers, toys, and any other object you might want to put in the vagina, bigger is not always better.

POSITIONING

You can play with the Thumb Love technique in almost any position: Stand at Attention, Spread Eagle, Gimme More, Lie Back and Take It, Swing Set, or Face Down, Bum Up!

TECHNIQUE

- Lube up your thumbs and brush them against her juicy lips.
- Once she's relaxed, insert your right thumb facing upward and press it against her upper vaginal wall. Only insert it as far as your first knuckle.
- As you press on the upper wall, pull your thumb out and curl it upward in a U motion to stroke her clitoral head.
- Repeat this scooping motion, resting your other fingers on her mons as you stroke.
- Remember to tell her how warm and sexy it feels to be inside of her!

VARIATIONS AND ADVANCED TECHNIQUES

- As you scoop upward with your right thumb, use your left thumb (with your palm facing down) to gently press and scoop against her lower vaginal wall.
- Once you've coordinated the scooping movement with both thumbs, try inserting your tongue into her vagina between them.

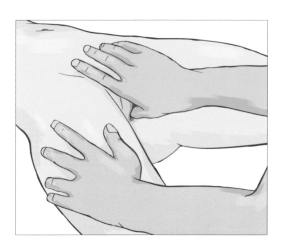

DR. JESS SUGGESTS . . .

Our obsession with size tends to focus on the penis, but vaginal size matters, too, and it's really more about finding the perfect fit (like a shoe!) than picking the biggest or smallest one you can find. One study that used MRI to examine the vaginal canal found that the average resting length from the entrance of the vagina to the cervix is less than 2½ inches (6.4 centimeters). However, there is extra space on each side of the cervix, and as she becomes sexually excited, this length increases as the cervix tents up—all the more reason to get her even more hot and bothered before you slip inside of her!

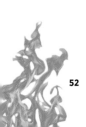

ALL ABOUT U

You've probably heard of the G-spot and the A-spot (and if you haven't, you will shortly). But can you find the U-spot? It's a small patch of sensitive tissues in the shape of an upside-down U that surrounds the urethra. Be sure to check it out!

POSITIONING
Play with the U-spot with your pretty lady while she's in the Gimme More position.

TECHNIQUE
- Use your fingers to separate the inner lips and reveal the shiny area where you'll find the urethral opening (pee hole) just above the vaginal opening.
- Use a wet finger, a tongue, or a vibrating toy to trace an upside-down U around the urethra.
- Press your lips right up against her vestibule, the area between the inner lips where you'll find the openings to the urethra and vagina, and create some wet suction while you run your tongue from side to side.

VARIATIONS AND ADVANCED TECHNIQUES
- While you're down there, use your tongue to trace and kiss all around Hart's line—the line that surrounds the vulval vestibule on the inside of the inner lips. If you leave the light on, you'll be able to see the difference between the matte skin of the vulva and the shinier skin of the vulval vestibule.
- If you're using your fingers, ask her to suck on them first to get them nice and wet.
- If you can practice a bit of self-control, you may even want to rub some lube on the tip of your penis and rub it all around her U-spot as an exhilarating tease.

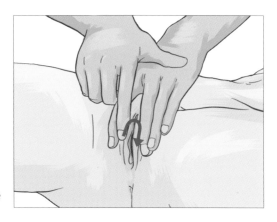

EXTENSION MOVE: THE NOSE JOB
- While you're eating out her tasty pussy, get your nose right in there and get messy. Sex is supposed to be wet and a little sloppy, so don't hold back.
- Use your nose to press gently against her clitoral head or stroke it through the hood.
- Run your nose along the groove between her lips.
- Use your hands to open up her labia and slide your lubed-up nose right into her vaginal opening as you breathe in and tell her how much you love it!

DR. JESS SUGGESTS . . .
The nose is an erogenous zone for many people, and its inner lining actually swells during sexual arousal much like the genitals and the breasts do.

COME HITHER

Make her purr by playfully petting the spongy tissue on the upper wall of her vagina. Known as the G-spot, this sexy area is located on the stomach-side wall of the vagina, about 2 to 3 inches (5 to 7.5 cm) from the entrance. Women (and sexologists!) love this move, because it serves as a reminder that deeper is not always better.

POSITIONING

Ask her to lie on her back in the Gimme More position and kneel between her spread legs.

TECHNIQUE

- Apply some lube to your index finger and play around, spreading her labia and planting kisses between her legs.
- Once she's worked up, insert your index finger with your palm facing upward. When you've buried your finger as deep as your second knuckle, curl it up in a "come hither" motion.
- If you feel a ridgelike area on the upper wall of her vagina, you've probably found her G-spot.
- As you curl your finger against this area, it may become firmer and the ridges may feel more prominent.

VARIATIONS AND ADVANCED TECHNIQUES

- The G-spot is sometimes described as the female prostate, so if you want to double your pleasure, lie on your sides next to each other and have her reach around to massage your prostate.

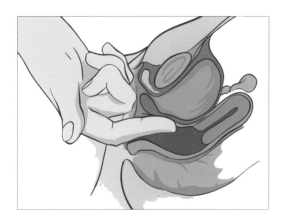

- Alternate the "come hither" gesture using your finger, tongue, and a vibrating toy.
- Use your thumb to play with her clitoris while you make the "come hither" motion with your index finger.

VARIATION: THE TICK TOCK

Try the Tick Tock technique to stimulate a larger area and make her scream your name (in a good way)! Women who enjoy G-spot stimulation report that the Tick Tock can lead to orgasm quickly.

TECHNIQUE

- Lube up your index and middle fingers and insert them into her pussy with your palm facing upward.
- Sweep your fingers back and forth against her upper vaginal wall in a tick-tock motion while you look her in the eyes with fierce intensity.

DR. JESS SUGGESTS . . .

Because the G-spot swells during arousal, it may be easier to recognize as she gets more turned on. Although researchers believe that every woman has a G-spot, it is not necessarily a hot spot for every woman, so be sure to ask for feedback if you're exploring new territory.

JUST RIGHT

The clitoris really is a thing of wonder, and it deserves some special attention during sex play. But sometimes direct stimulation of the head can be too much to handle, so Just Right can come in handy as a way to make it smile and tingle in all the right ways.

POSITIONING

Kneel over her chest while she assumes the Lie Back and Take It position. You should be facing toward her feet and may want to place some pillows beside her hips as supports for your hands.

TECHNIQUE

- Place your middle finger on the hood of her clitoris facing toward her feet. Make sure the tip of your finger lines up with the edge of her hood while the rest of it presses against her mound.
- Pull up on her hood to reveal the shiny head of the clitoris and lean down to breathe some warm air over it with wide-open lips. Change the shape of your lips and purse them to let out some cool direct air.
- Trace seductive ovals with your tongue all around the area without making direct contact with the head.
- Pull up and down on the hood and venus mound to stroke the clitoral shaft as you breathe over the clitoral pearl.

VARIATIONS AND ADVANCED TECHNIQUES

- Reach around and pull up on the clitoral hood during intercourse in the doggie-style position.
- Pair the Just Right with the Cross My Fingers technique (page 47).

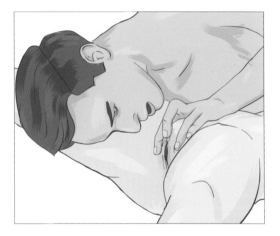

DR. JESS SUGGESTS . . .

During the plateau phase of sexual arousal, the clitoral head may actually appear to retract into the hood as its sensitivity increases. Some women love a whole lot of clitoral rubbing while others like the indirect stimulation afforded by some rhythmic hood stroking. Ask her to touch herself so you can watch and learn, or get her to take you by the hand and show you how she likes it.

THE DARING ELEVATOR

Have you noticed that the most intense orgasms often follow a long period of sex play? It's no surprise: Prolonged arousal and plateau phases can lead to intensified pleasure and stronger, longer orgasms. Use the Daring Elevator technique to work her up very gradually and promote a full-body orgasm.

POSITIONING

Ask her to lie in the Swing Set position and relax with her eyes closed—or blindfold her.

TECHNIQUE

- Sensually caress her whole body, beginning with her feet and working your way up to her inner thighs. Once you've reached her thighs, move up to her face and work your way back down to her hips so that you're drawing awareness and blood flow to her pelvic region.
- As you caress her body, try a "spider pull" stroke: Start with all five fingertips resting lightly against her skin and pull your fingertips together to meet in the center.
- Play with a warm-up technique or two (e.g., the Finger Lick or the Vee-Jay-Jay) to get her excited and yearning for more.
- Encourage her to breathe deeply and think of a hot fantasy or dream that turns her on.
- Begin the Daring Elevator by very gently pressing your middle finger against the opening of her vagina without letting it slip inside. Press and release as slowly as possible 10 to 12 times to promote circulation to the area and help build up her orgasmic platform.
- Maintaining a slow rhythm, slip your fingers into her vagina only until you reach your first knuckle and slide in and out another 10 to 12 times. If she thrusts against you, try to adjust your movements to control the depth of penetration so that you don't go past your first knuckle.
- Increase the depth of penetration to reach your second knuckle and continue to finger her with another 10 to 12 slow insertions.

- Finally, insert your finger as slowly as you can all the way up to your third knuckle. Feel her warmth wrap around you as you gradually increase your fingering speed, taking cues from the movements of her hips.

VARIATIONS AND ADVANCED TECHNIQUES

- Add your index finger into the mix if she likes a little more girth.
- Try the Daring Elevator using your penis during intercourse. This type of slow sex requires a ton of self-control, but it can lead to unbelievably intense orgasms for both of you!
- If she enjoys multiple orgasms, try this technique between orgasms to tease her a little and continue building tension.

DR. JESS SUGGESTS . . .

Most of us have a tendency to rush through sex, because it's just so exciting and satisfying. And though quickies can sometimes do the trick, a recent study found that most men and women actually want a full 18 minutes of foreplay—all the fun stuff other than intercourse. So take your time and enjoy the ride! Whatever your inclination may be with regard to speed, slow down by at least 50 percent because we have a natural tendency to rush when we get nervous or excited.

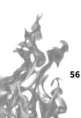

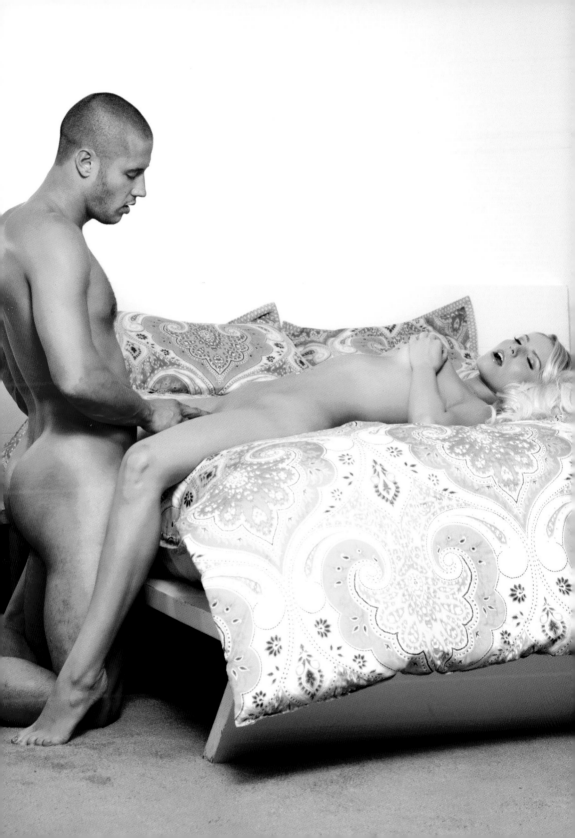

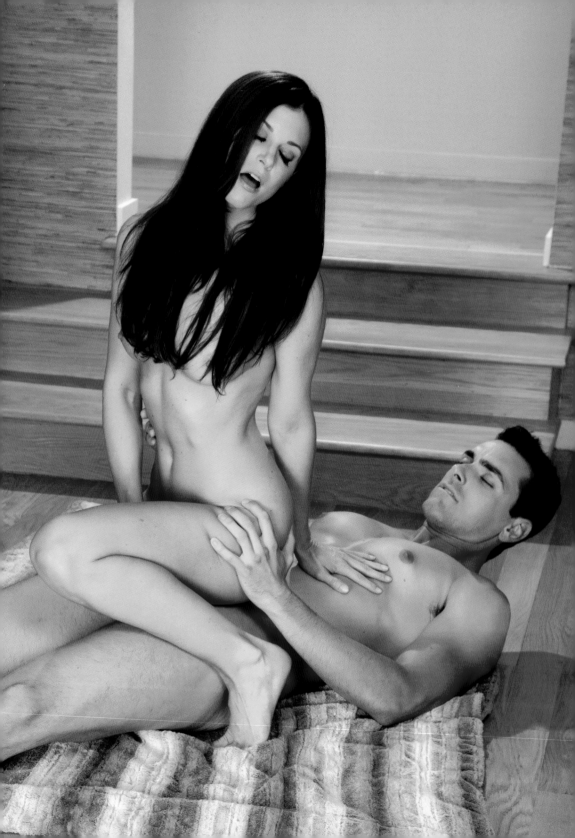

CHAPTER 4

THE HOTTEST TECHNIQUES FOR MIND-BLOWING ORGASMS

MAKE HER WEAK IN THE KNEES and satiate her burning desire with these finishing moves designed to make her orgasmic experience one (or more) that she'll never forget! Whether she's a screamer, a squirter, or a squirmer, she's sure to love at least a few of these take-her-over-the-edge techniques. So don't wait for a rainy day to try them out—read on and get started!

Bear in mind that orgasms cover a huge range of experiences. Some women describe their orgasms as:

- Relaxing
- Cathartic
- Earth-shattering
- Mind-blowing
- Nice
- Shaky
- Smooth
- Scary
- Exciting
- Underwhelming
- Overwhelming
- Relieving
- Unreal
- Feverish
- Wet
- Exhilarating
- Soothing

Each of these experiences can be equally pleasurable; a relaxing orgasm can be just as memorable and satisfying as an earth-shattering one. From gentle tremble to thunderous tremor, take the time to enjoy both the erotic journey and the wondrous destination.

SWEET PINCH

This move lets you play with control and stimulates the two areas most associated with female orgasm: the G-spot and the clitoral head.

POSITIONING

Kneel between her legs as she leans back against the headboard in the Gimme More position.

TECHNIQUE

- Start by gently inserting your index finger into her vagina and curl it upward to rub the G-spot on the upper wall. If she likes it, stroke slowly and gently to tease her a little.
- As she gets more worked up, press your thumb over her clitoral hood or pearl, pinching your thumb and index finger together as you pull in and out.

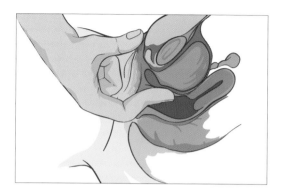

VARIATIONS AND ADVANCED TECHNIQUES

Use three wet fingers of your spare hand to draw a figure eight over her perineum while you pinch her sweetly. Slip your tongue into her vagina below your index finger and twirl it around against her vaginal walls as they fill with blood and become firmer.

DR. JESS SUGGESTS . . .

The sensitivity of her erogenous zones will vary during her sexual response cycle. During the arousal and plateau stages, her hot spots may be more sensitive to touch, so be sure to ask her if she wants more or less pressure. Conversely, as she approaches orgasm, you may be able to apply firmer pressure, as the release of endorphins may give her a feeling of euphoria and increase her pain threshold.

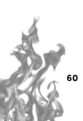

THE HUMAN VIBRATOR

You don't need batteries or remote controls to get her private parts buzzing. Just use your vocal cords and some firm pressure to mimic the vibrating sensations of her favorite toy.

POSITIONING

Anything goes for the human vibrator, but the Lie Back and Take It position is a popular favorite.

TECHNIQUE

- Run your tongue along the crease between her thighs and her venus mound as you work your way down to her pussy.
- Open your mouth nice and wide and use your lips to create suction around her vulva as you suck away.
- Begin moaning or making a buzzing sound as you suck to create a vibrating sensation.
- Move your tongue up to her clitoral pearl and continue "vibrating" as you suck away.

VARIATIONS AND ADVANCED TECHNIQUES

Does she love powerful vibrations? Wear a vibrating cock ring on your tongue when you're going down on her.

DR. JESS SUGGESTS . . .

Vibrators are popular with women, men, and couples. More than half of American women have used a vibrator, and research suggests that those who do use vibrators report higher levels of sexual satisfaction.

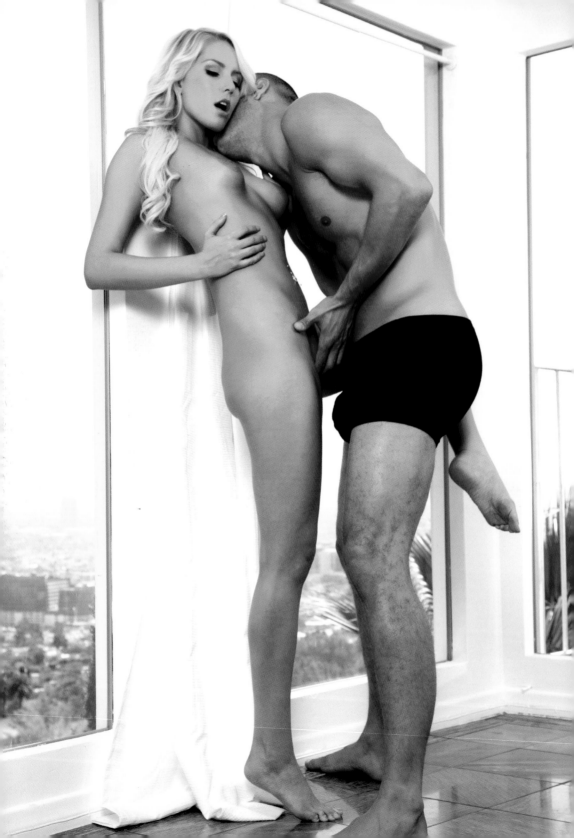

THE SPRINKLER

The Sprinkler builds upon the Sweet Pinch (page 60) to create more friction and pressure against the urethral sponge and encourage her to release her sweet love juices. Let's begin with a strong reminder that squirting isn't a sideshow act, and only some women report experiences of ejaculation. It will likely only detract from your sexual pleasure if ejaculation becomes a goal, but if she likes the feeling of letting go and getting wet, then give the Sprinkler a try. Remember that G-spot pleasure is subjective: Just like a foot rub, some women love it and others find it uncomfortable. Encourage her to try touching this area on her own before you play with the Sprinkler.

POSITIONING

Kneel between her legs as she assumes the Stand at Attention or Gimme More position.

TECHNIQUE

- Get her all riled up, and then insert your middle and ring fingers into her wet vagina and press upward against the top wall.
- Stroke the upper wall with both fingers, curling upward in an in-and-out motion while your thumb presses against her clitoral hood and pubic mound.
- As you feel the upper wall (G-spot area) become firmer and more ridged, press down on her abdomen just above her venus mound with your other hand.
- Continue stroking rhythmically at a fairly fast pace, applying firm pressure and encouraging her to let go and relax.
- If she wants to experiment with ejaculation, she may want to bear down with her pelvic floor muscles as opposed to tensing up.

DR. JESS SUGGESTS . . .

Female ejaculate is expelled through the urethra (pee hole) and is similar to male prostatic fluids. Don't worry—it's not just pee. As in the case of men, sometimes ejaculation and orgasm occur simultaneously, and sometimes they are separate experiences. For some women, ejaculation can be intensely pleasurable and evident, while for others their experience may range from discomfort to indifference. Ejaculation can even go unnoticed during sex play. Each of these experiences is normal and healthy. To ease concerns about peeing during sex play, simply empty your bladder beforehand and rest assured that if a little pee is released, it's no big deal at all.

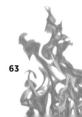

THE AFICIONADO

The Aficionado loves the female form and relishes in the art of going down. He loves the taste, smell, texture, temperature, and aura of the beautiful vulva and expresses this passion through movement, breath, and sound.

POSITIONING

Since this technique is really all about you, find a comfortable position that will allow you to flexibly move your face, lips, hands, and any other body part you'd like to rub up against her pussy. The Director's Chair may be most practical, because you can move around to access her sweet goods from several angles.

TECHNIQUE

- French kiss her and tell her how much you love the way her lips feel.
- Keep kissing her, tracing a sloppy, wet line of kisses down the center of her body until you reach her venus mound.
- Dive into her vulva with your lips, tongue, nose, cheeks, and chin. Eat, suck, kiss, lick, and slurp away, letting out heavy moans and breaths to show your pleasure. Appreciate eating her out the way you would taste a fine wine, cognac, or rich dessert.

- Look up into her eyes and tell her how much you like it. (See below for some dirty-talk tips.)
- Then tell her *why* you love it. After all, you *are* the Aficionado.
- Be sure to keep breathing her in, letting out excited exhalations, and looking up to her with a stare that screams, "I just can't get enough of you."

These dirty lines may help you get started:
- "I love the way you taste."
- "I love the smell!"
- "I can't get enough."
- "You're so warm and beautiful."
- "I want to suck you dry!"
- "Shove your pussy/cookie/goods (insert her favorite word here) in my face!"
- "You make me so hard."
- "You're all I ever wanted."
- "You're juicy and delicious."
- "I feel safe between your legs."
- "I can't resist you."
- "I love putting my face in your pussy, because it tastes so sweet."
- "You're the only one for me."
- "You taste so good, I'd pay for this."

DR. JESS SUGGESTS . . .

Many women have been taught that their vulvas and vaginas are unclean and smelly, when nothing could be farther from the truth for most healthy women because the vagina really is like a self-cleaning oven. As for its natural odors, they are usually quite mild, and many men report feeling aroused by the scent of vaginal secretions. If you're one of these men, be sure to let your partner know, because it may help her lie back, relax, and enjoy the ride.

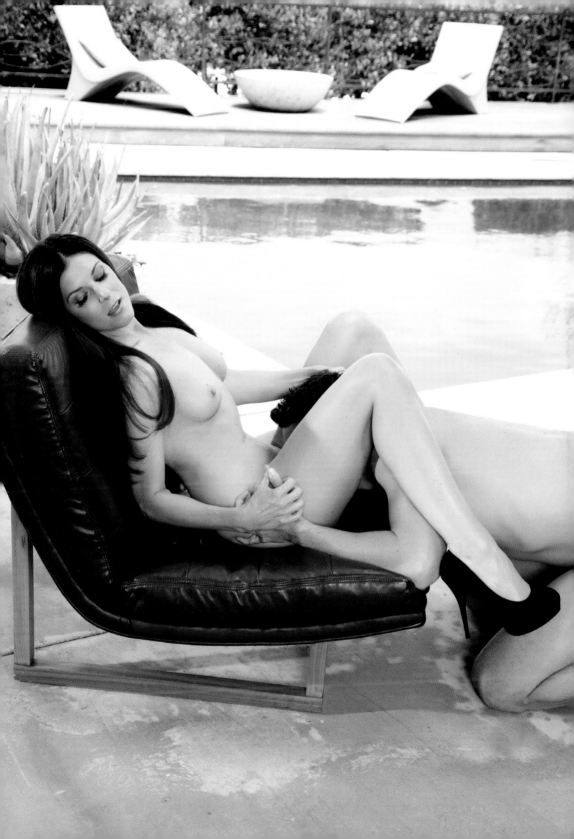

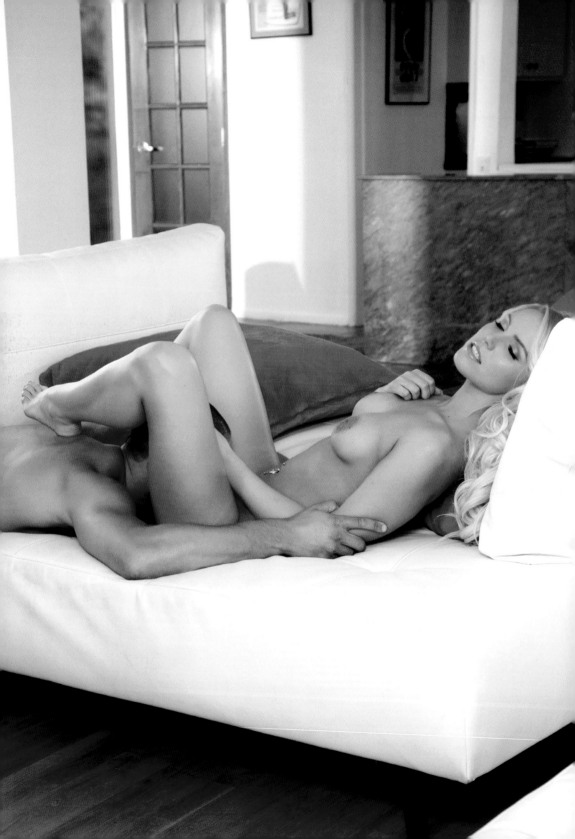

LIP LOCK

She may not be the type to kiss and tell, but the Lip Lock is a technique that has women talking!

POSITIONING

Try the Lip Lock with your partner lying on her back with one hip propped up with a few pillows. Assume the Lusty T position and have her throw one leg over your back.

TECHNIQUE

- Get your lips nice and wet with your saliva or your favorite flavored lube.
- Use your lips to gently squeeze her inner labia together and then run your tongue between the groove you've created.
- Breathe in and out heavily as you stroke with your tongue.

VARIATIONS AND ADVANCED TECHNIQUES

- Try alternating among in-and-out, up-and-down, and side-to-side motions with your tongue.
- Suck away as you run your tongue between the groove of her labia. Tell her how much you enjoy the natural sounds and tastes.

DR. JESS SUGGESTS . . .

Your mouth is one of your hottest and most sensitive erogenous zones, so enjoy the sensation of pressing your lips against her warm, wet labia. When you kiss, your brain releases a frenzy of sexual energy as it sends messages to the rest of your body's sexual system, including your tongue, skin, and genitals.

BAD MANNERS

Forget about social conventions that frown on talking with your mouth full. They obviously don't apply while muff diving. Let your big mouth and loose lips get you into the kind of trouble that demands a good punishing!

POSITIONING
Anything goes!

TECHNIQUE

- While enjoying your regular weekday dinner, interrupt the meal with some saucy compliments: "Your butt looks so hot in those pants" or "I want to tear your clothes off!"
- Get up from the table and carry her over to the couch or another soft surface before removing her bottoms.
- Put your face between her legs and lick, suck, and rub all over while telling her about all the things you want to do to her:
    - "I want to make you come."
    - "I'm going to make you scream."
    - "I want to make your breasts tingle."
    - "I want to make you weak in the knees."
    - "I want to taste your cum."

VARIATIONS AND ADVANCED TECHNIQUES

Take her by the hand and have her touch herself as you eat her out so that she gets the exact rhythm, speed, and pressure she is craving.

DR. JESS SUGGESTS . . .

The brain really is our biggest sex organ, so if you can tap into your lady's fantasies with some sexy talk, it can be way hotter than anything you can do with your hands or lips. If you have trouble getting started with talking dirty, just begin with sexy compliments about her body or her skills as a lover. Start slowly and be sure to take some time to talk about your feelings and reactions to the things you both said in the heat of the moment after the sex session is over.

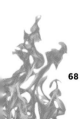

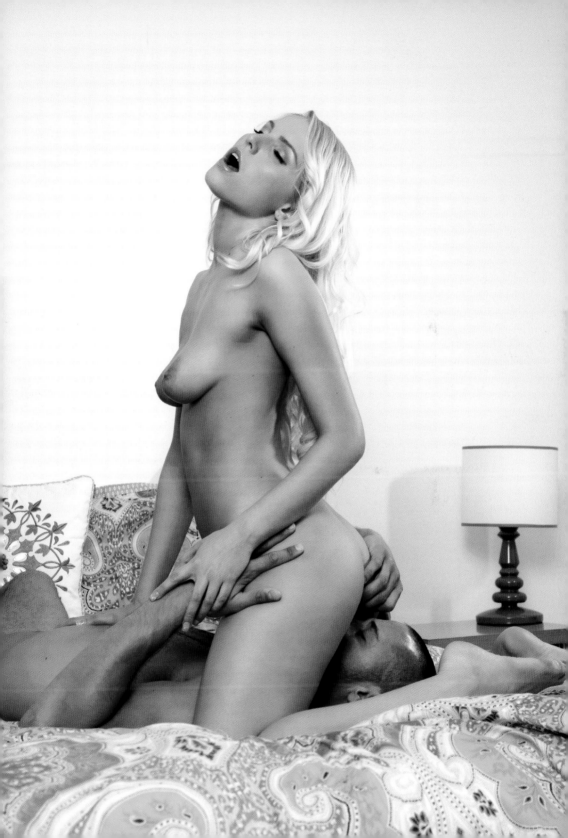

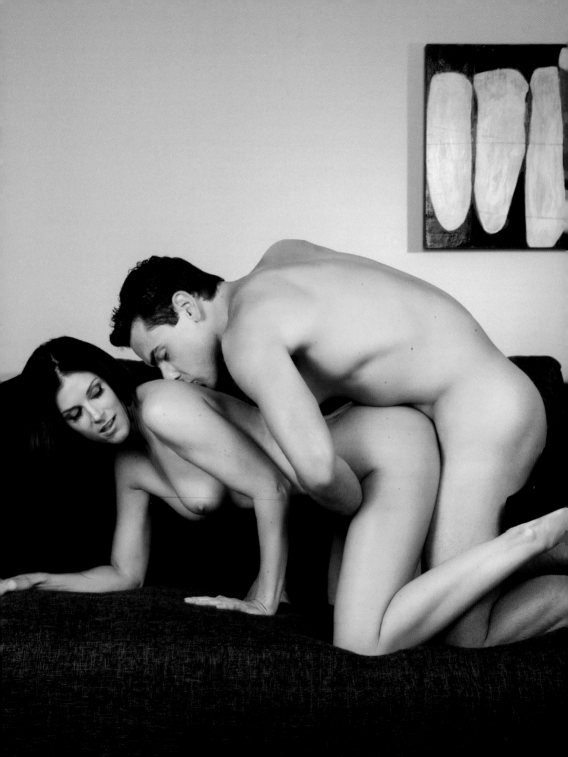

◀ THE HOT BUTTON

Most women don't want you to treat her clitoris like an elevator button as soon as you discover its not-so-secret location, but a little pulsing at the onset of orgasm can lead to more intense, longer-lasting orgasms.

POSITIONING

Use the Hot Button in any position that allows you to reach her clitoral pearl with your thumb.

TECHNIQUE

- Play with her body and encourage her to fantasize about her hottest sex dream until she is approaching orgasm.
- As she comes close to climaxing, pulse your wet thumb against her clitoral pearl rhythmically in one-second intervals.

VARIATIONS AND ADVANCED TECHNIQUES

Use the Hot Button during intercourse to take her over the edge and make her orgasms even more intense. You can reach around from behind in the Dog position, or access her with a free hand while she rides you.

THE TONGUE TWISTER

If you're a bit of a chatterbox, all those years of exercising your tongue are finally going to pay off. Use the Tongue Twister to tantalize her pussy and leave her *beyond* speechless.

POSITIONING

Any position will do, but if she's a squirmer, lie between her legs as she assumes the Gimme More position and hold her knees steady with your hands.

TECHNIQUE

- Begin by licking all around her thighs and vulva with a very sloppy tongue. Suck it all in and breathe heavily so that she knows you like it.
- Once she's worked up, thrust your tongue into her wet pussy with your mouth wide open. Run your tongue around inside of her in a wide circle, pressing into the walls of her vagina.

- Switch directions and continue sucking with your wet lips.

VARIATIONS AND ADVANCED TECHNIQUES

Try twirling your tongue in a figure eight shape.

THE TUBE OF LOVE

Roll your tongue into a firm tube before wrapping it around her sweet spots to make her moan. You may have heard that the ability to roll your tongue is hereditary, but this is actually an inaccurate oversimplification. To learn to roll your tongue, purse your lips tightly and try to push your tongue out while rolling the sides in toward one another. If you really can't roll your tongue, fret not! You can pinch the sides of your tongue together with your fingers to create an equally sexy tube.

POSITIONING

Have your partner assume the Swing Set position and kneel on a pillow between her legs.

TECHNIQUE

- Practice rolling your tongue into a tube and run it in and out of your mouth as you breathe some warm, moist air over her thighs and venus mound.
- Use a finger or two to pull up on her clitoral hood so that the pearl is slightly exposed, and slide your Tube of Love back and forth over it as you lightly tickle your fingers all over her labia with your spare hand.
- Work your way down to her vagina and slide the Tube of Love in and out while keeping your hands busy with her labia and perineum.

VARIATIONS AND ADVANCED TECHNIQUES

- While you thrust in and out with the Tube of Love, tickle your nose against her clitoral pearl.
- Try this technique on your back in the Sit on My Face position.

DR. JESS SUGGESTS . . .

If she loves the sensation of the Tube of Love, use it to entice her outside of the bedroom and eroticize your relationship. While you're out in public, give her a playful sneak peek of what's to come later by slipping a tiny bit of your rolled tongue out from between your lips when she least expects it. Lean over and whisper, "Later..." or "You like that?" in her ear to build her excitement. Anticipation is hot and both her brain and her body will respond as you trigger the memory of the last time she experienced your Tube of Love!

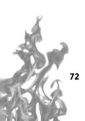

THE THREE-WAY

This is a sure-fire finishing move that will launch her orgasms into overdrive.

POSITIONING

Do whatever you can to get in between her legs with easy access to both her clitoral pearl and her butt hole. It may be most comfortable to kneel between her legs in the Swing Set position, but you may have to improvise depending on which moves you begin with.

TECHNIQUE

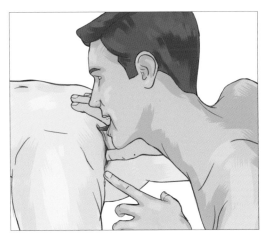

- As she approaches orgasm, start stroking the shaft and pearl of her clitoris with the firm tip of your tongue.
- Continue the clitoral tongue-stroking and slide your thumb in and out of her pussy, maintaining pressure against the upper vaginal wall.
- Use the index finger of your other hand (with lots of lube) to apply firm pressure to her bum hole and trace a smooth line from her anus to her fourchette along her perineum.
- Increase the speed and pressure, maintaining a constant rhythm between both hands and your tongue.

VARIATIONS AND ADVANCED TECHNIQUES

- If she isn't up for bum play, simply pay more attention to her perineum.
- Replace the smooth strokes of both hands with circular motions or figure eights.

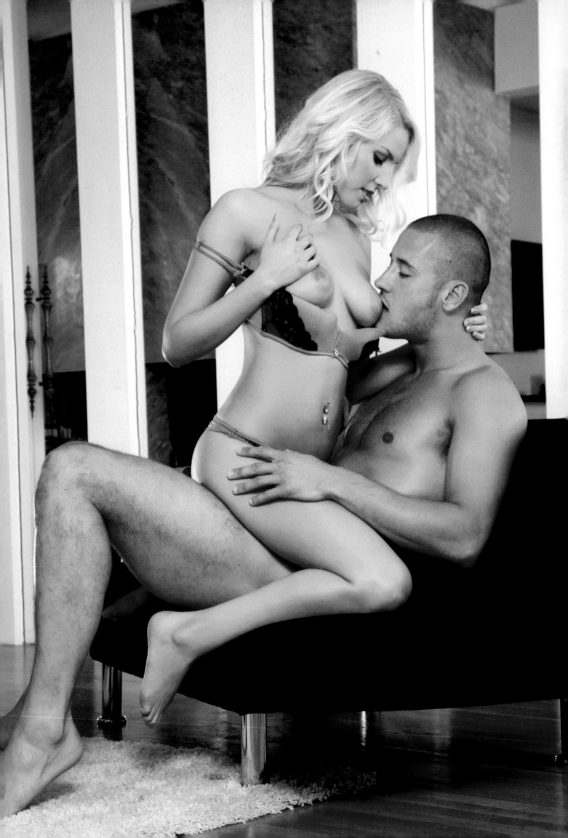

CHAPTER 5

HIS SWEET SPOTS: MALE ANATOMY AND EROGENOUS ZONES

BRIMMING WITH SEXUAL ENERGY, the male genitals are also things of wonder that can literally bring you to your knees. Have fun exploring and getting to know his most intimate and electrical parts!

The penis is actually a complex organ and varies greatly from man to man in terms of shape, size, color, curvature, and sensitivity. Over time, each penis evolves and its hot spots and responsiveness are redefined. This means that exploring his hot spots and gauging his reactions is not a one-shot deal. Even if you think you know a penis inside out, it's always good to get back to basics every couple of months to learn about its new sweets spots and sensitivities.

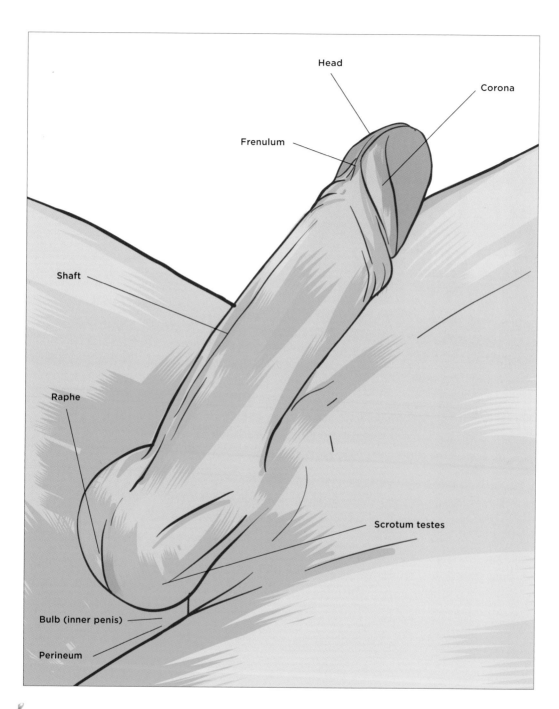

Head

Corona

Frenulum

Shaft

Raphe

Scrotum testes

Bulb (inner penis)

Perineum

PENIS PARTS

Head: This sexy topper is the most innervated part of the penis.

Shaft: The main event connects the head to the base and scrotum. It fills with blood during erection.

Bulb: This is an often-overlooked frenzy zone that can take the male orgasm to new heights! Located inside the body, it can be stimulated through the perineum. MRI imaging shows that the penis boomerangs in shape during intercourse, and its deepest point may just be the hot zone you've been searching for.

Corona: This delicious ridge surrounds the base of the head and swells with pride if you're nice to it.

Frenulum: What a hot spot! This is the little piece of connective tissue on the underside of the penis at the top of the shaft and base of the head.

Foreskin: This protective layer of skin that covers the head of the penis is sometimes removed by parents when the man is still a baby through a process called circumcision.

Testes: Contained within the scrotal sac, these boys—also known as the balls—are a stronghold of sizzling virility.

Scrotum: This sac contains the testes.

Perineum: The supersensitive space between the anus and the base of the scrotum through which you can stimulate the mysterious bulb of the penis and the prostate, the perineum is also believed to be the location of the "million-dollar point" located at its very back in front of the anal opening.

Anus: This is the butt hole. Some men love to have their butt hole played with on the outside, some love to be penetrated (often with extra special attention paid to the prostate), and others like to keep their anus a safe distance away from all foreign objects. To each his own, but bear in mind that personal anal preference is entirely unrelated to sexual orientation. (See page 136 for more on anal play.)

Prostate: Just like the female G-spot, the prostate is located inside the male body and can be accessed through the anus on its upper wall.

Raphe: The dividing line that runs from the underside of the penis all the way back to the anus, crossing over the scrotal sac and perineum.

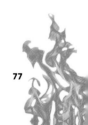

ALL ABOUT HIS ORGASM

Male sexual response is often dumbed-down in our culture; there is an erroneous assumption that all men are simple sexual beings. But this is not the case! Men are just as varied, complex, and unique as women are sexually, and they require both physical and mental stimulation to enjoy mind-blowing sex.

Just like women, men can experience a range of physical responses to sexual stimuli with or without the desired mental responses. So getting your head into the red-hot game of sex is just as important for men. This four-stage model outlines some of the physical changes that men may experience during sexual response.

Bear in mind that the body acts in mysterious ways, so these sensations and reactions can occur independently of one another and in a nonsequential fashion. For example, we've all heard of the good old NRB—the No Reason Boner—right? Sometimes penises decide to get rock hard for no good reason, and other times they decide they're not up for an erection even though the rest of the body is ready to get frisky.

DESIRE AND AROUSAL

- Thoughts turn to sex, intimacy, romance, eroticism, and physical connection.
- Heart rate, breathing, and blood pressure increase.
- Nipples fill will blood and become enlarged.
- Muscles tense up.
- Penis fills with blood, grows, and hardens.
- Drops of precum may be expelled from the penis through the urethra.
- Skin may become flushed.
- Testicles swell and the scrotum tightens.

INTENSE AROUSAL

- Breathing and heart rate continue to increase.
- The body perspires.
- Testes draw up into the scrotum, making it feel "tighter."
- Muscle tension increases.

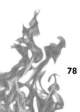

ORGASM

- Muscles spasm or tense up involuntarily.
- Blood pressure, breathing, and heart rate increase.
- Toes curl.
- PC muscle and anal sphincter contract.
- Rhythmic contractions of the prostate, perineal muscles, and shaft may be followed by ejaculation of fluid from the urethra.
- Various natural sounds may emanate from his lips.
- Sexual tension is released.

POSTORGASM

- Heart rate, blood pressure, and breathing slow to regular levels
- The erect penis returns to its previous size.
- Most men experience a refractory, or rest, period after orgasm during. This period can range from a few minutes to several days, but the fun doesn't have to stop after orgasm. Even if the penis needs a rest, there are plenty of fun tricks and techniques that men can pull off *sans* penis using hands, lips, breath, and tongue.

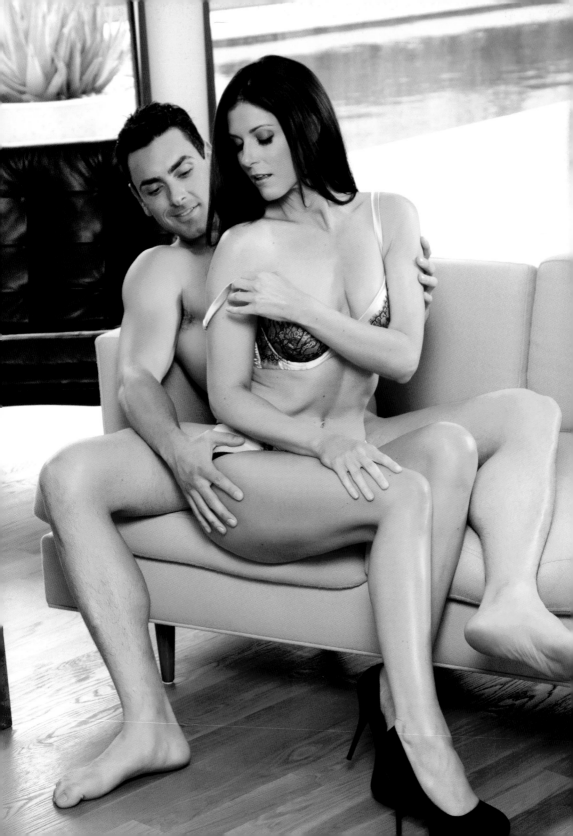

CHAPTER 6

HOT MOVES TO RILE HIM UP

BE THE SULTRY SEDUCTRESS EVERY MAN DREAMS OF by getting him all worked up with these sizzling-hot starter moves. It may be hard to resist grabbing his throbbing manhood as soon as it begins to stir, but taking your time to rev up his engine allows you to develop a deeper connection and makes his body ache for more of your smoldering hot touch.

If he's still dressed when you're just getting started, look him in the eye while you run your fingers inside his waistband to whet his appetite. And if he's one of those guys who gets butt naked as soon as he walks in the door, take him by the hands and guide his fingers to a warm spot between your legs as you stroke your fingertips against the small of his back.

Don't try to use all of these moves in one sitting—that would be exhausting! And besides, you want to tease and tantalize him, not torture the poor man. Choose one or two that you feel most confident experimenting with and start from there before moving on to the hotter moves in the next section. You'll be able to gauge his response by his facial expressions, pelvic movements, and changes in breathing.

And though these techniques are designed to get him in the mood initially, you can always go back to them later on in the sex session if you want to slow things down or make his hard-on last longer for your personal use and enjoyment.

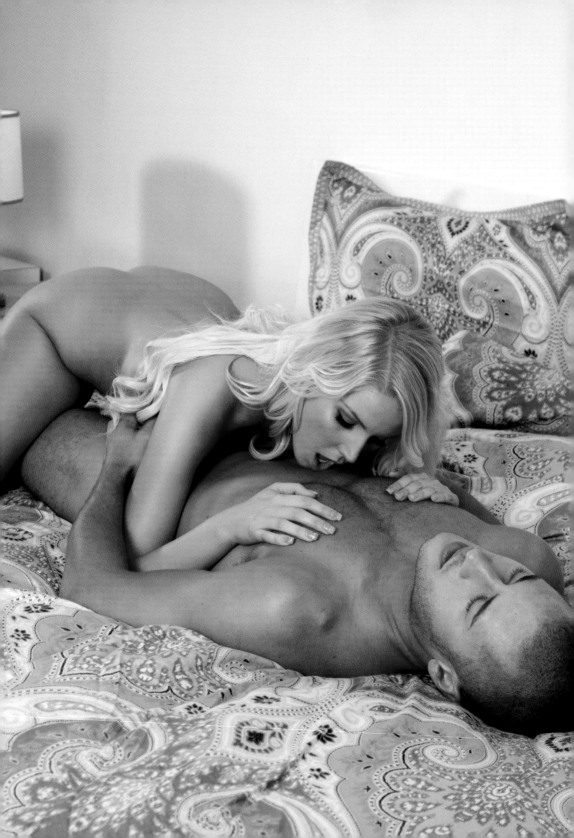

◀ THE HOT TRACE

Want to tease him a little and make him beg for more? Then try the Hot Trace to make him ache for more of your tantalizing tongue's talent.

POSITIONING

Have your man lie on his back while you straddle his thighs.

TECHNIQUE

- Begin at his nipples and use your tongue to trace circles around the outer edges of his areolae.
- Work your way down to his pelvic area with your tongue and lick his abdomen all around his penis. Trace a line around its outer edge from base to tip, allowing some incidental contact with his shaft and head.

VARIATIONS AND ADVANCED TECHNIQUES

Extend your trace all the way down to his thighs as you draw a warm, wet line around his balls and tell him how big they feel against your tongue.

THE LICKING HAND

Your tongue can work wonders on his member, but you have ten titillating fingers that can do so much more with the right amount of pressure and lube! Your fingers are not only more agile than your tongue, but they also come in handy when the mood strikes you in more public places. Try the Licking Hand to spark his interest while you're on the road and can't justify climbing under the table or onto the sticky movie theater floor.

POSITIONING

Any position goes for the Licking Hand!

TECHNIQUE

- Warm up your fingers and get them soaking wet with lube.
- Use your index and middle finger to "lick" all around his shaft, alternating slow winding motions with quick, short lines.
- Add another hand (index and middle finger or one big flat palm) to simulate two tongues.
- As you "lick" away with your hands, tell him how good it feels and ask him if he'd like to have two women licking his throbbing shaft.

VARIATIONS AND ADVANCED TECHNIQUES

If your position allows for it, breathe heavily over your fingers as they lick away and add your real tongue to the mix so that it feels like he's being ravaged by a group of tongues.

THE TEASE

Men love sex! But the notion that every man is always raring to go at the drop of a dime is horribly inaccurate. Most men like to be seduced and enjoy some sexy teasing as a precursor to heavy sex play, so take your time to work him up and make him beg for more.

POSITIONING

Have your man lie on his back while you assume the Reverse Cowgirl position.

TECHNIQUE

- Arch your back as you lean down and breathe all over his thighs so that he gets a nice view from behind.
- Warm up your hands with some sexy massage oil or lube and give him a sensuous thigh massage using very slow, gentle strokes.
- Breathe all over his oiled-up skin and let the backs of your hands and inner wrists brush up against his penis and balls without allowing any purposeful contact.
- Tell him that if he behaves and is a patient gentleman, good things will come his way.

VARIATIONS AND ADVANCED TECHNIQUES

Try the Tease in other positions like Gimme More and the Director's Chair, using your breasts to massage his thighs instead of your hands.

DR. JESS SUGGESTS . . .

Playing with fantasies about threesomes or group sex can be unbelievably hot! Group sex is a top sex fantasy for both men and women, and many monogamous couples talk about these scenarios with no intention of living them out. However, it is important to talk to your partner about boundaries beforehand to make sure he or she is comfortable with this type of erotic talk. Debriefing and offering reassurance (e.g., "In real life, you're all I want! It's just fun to fantasize and talk about threesomes.") is also essential to a happy relationship and sex life. On the other hand, if you're up for acting out threesomes and group sex, that's perfectly okay, too! You just need to put considerable time and energy into preparing for your first experience to ensure that it is safe and pleasurable.

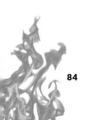

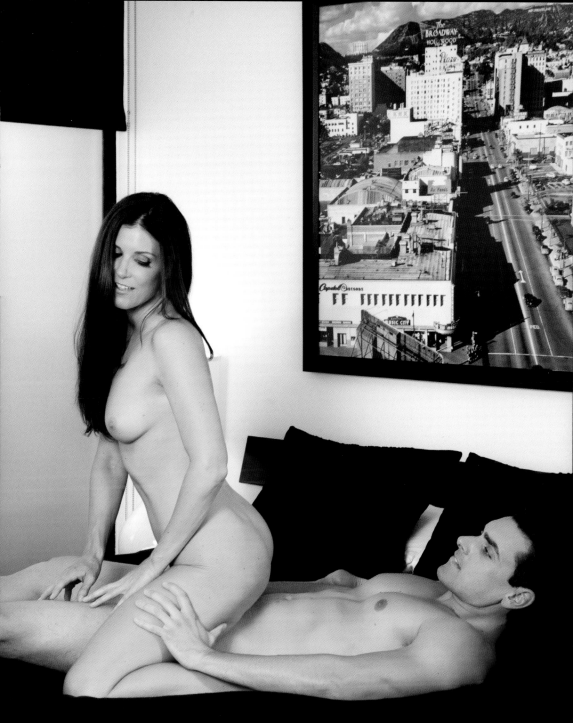

THE WET POLE DANCER

Want to get him hard and make him ache for more? Then dance your tongue around his cock as you look up into his eyes with a flirty gaze.

POSITIONING

Have your man lean back against the headboard of your bed or in a chair in the Gimme More position as you kneel between his legs.

TECHNIQUE

- Cup your breasts in your hands and ask him if he likes to watch.
- Use your tongue to lick all around his shaft, corona, and head, as if it were dancing on a pole.
- Move your tongue in different patterns to find out what makes him tick, and practice the motions on the thin skin of your inner wrist so the techniques will come naturally once things get steamy:
  - Barely there flicks of the tongue against the frenulum
  - Straight short lines
  - Long slow lines
  - Big, slow, snakelike S patterns
  - Zigzags
  - Figure eights
  - Heavy pulses with the flat underside of your tongue

VARIATIONS AND ADVANCED TECHNIQUES

Dance your tongue all around his balls while you stroke his shaft with a well-lubed hand.

DR. JESS SUGGESTS . . .

If he loves the Wet Pole Dancer, play with it in and out of the bedroom. Tease him while you're out for dinner with a little pre-show on your straw as you sip your drink. Better yet, dance your tongue around your fingers as you taste your dessert or tickle his finger with your breath and tongue in the car on the way home. Use subtle tongue strokes as you tease and look him in the eye flirtatiously. Don't exaggerate or overdo it, because you don't want to look like a porn star—just the sexiest version of yourself.

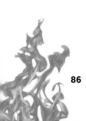

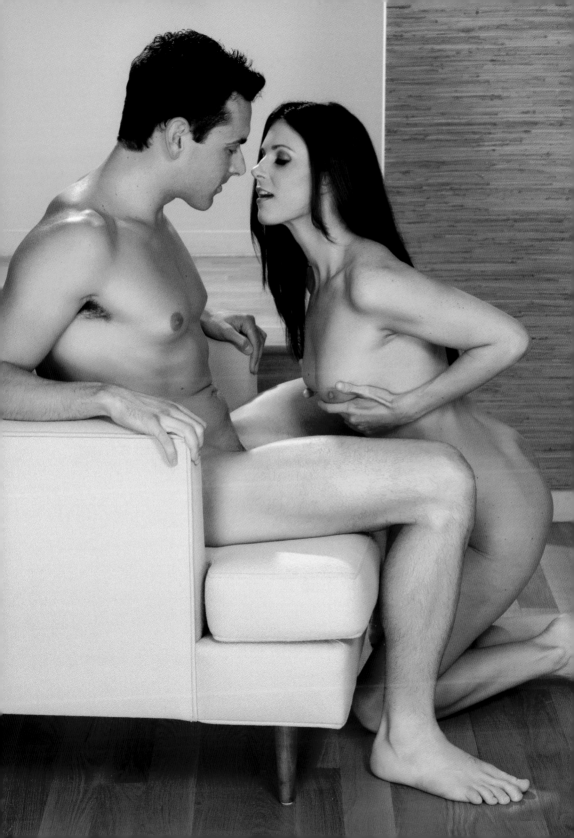

THE ONE-LANE HIGHWAY

The male body is full of erogenous zones, and the raphe—the dividing line that runs down the underside of the penis, over the scrotal sac, and through the perineum to the anus—is no exception. In fact, many men report coming to orgasm more quickly when their partner strokes the raphe of the perineum during intercourse and oral sex.

POSITIONING

Try this sensuous move in the Spread Eagle or Swing Set positions.

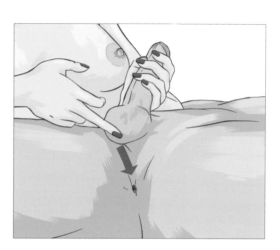

TECHNIQUE

- Trace a slow, sensuous line with a wet finger from the tip of his penis to his butt hole.
- Apply a bit of extra pressure to his frenulum and at the base of his penis before easing up as you cross over the center line of his balls and perineum.
- Retrace your line in the opposite direction and follow the wet line with your breath using pursed lips.

VARIATIONS AND ADVANCED TECHNIQUES

Use your tongue and a wet finger at the same time. Begin with your tongue at the tip of his penis and your finger against his butt hole and trace the lines toward one another, meeting in the middle of his scrotum.

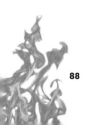

THE HARMONICA

The lower side of the penis deserves lots of extra attention! This is because the highly sensitive frenulum and the inner spongy region that fills with blood during an erection can be stimulated from the underside. Use the Harmonica to get him hard and make him sing with pleasure.

POSITIONING

Kneel next to your man in the the Lusty T as he relaxes on his back.

TECHNIQUE

- Press his penis upward against his abdomen using your thumb and index fingers.
- Run your lips and tongue up and down his entire cock. Moan to create some vibrations against his sensitive spots.
- Use your other hand, oiled with a generous amount of lube, to fondle his balls.

VARIATIONS AND ADVANCED TECHNIQUES

Although men don't generally like you to use teeth during oral sex, you can gently rub your upper front teeth against his shaft if you use lots of lube to do so. This can be very empowering for you if you like to play with dominance and submission, but it is best reserved for partners who have a good amount of trust and communication. Teeth usually have no place in a one-night stand.

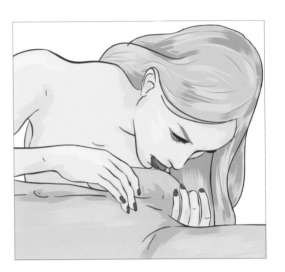

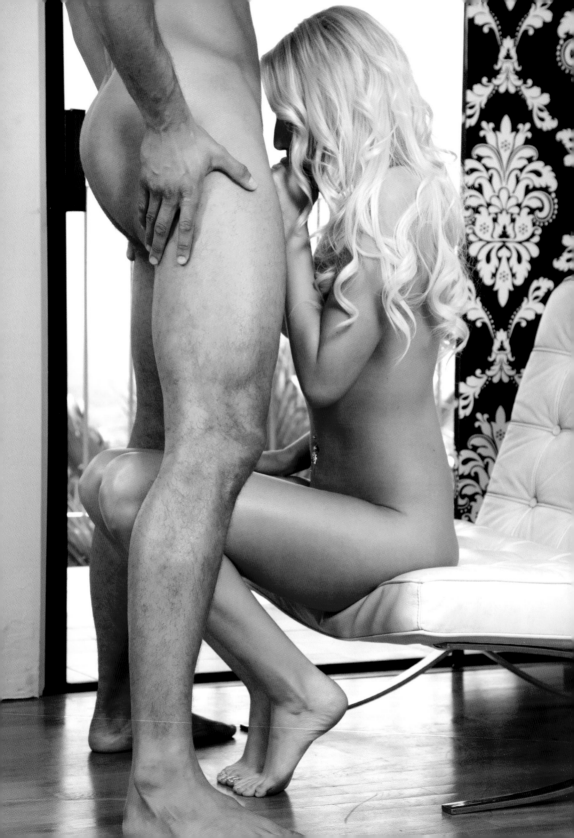

THE AIR HEAD

This is a great warm-up move for both of you! If you love giving head, it gives you a taste of what's to come while making him crave more of what your warm mouth has to offer.

POSITIONING

The Air Head works well with your man in the Stand at Attention position. You can kneel on the floor between his legs or sit on the edge of the bed.

DR. JESS SUGGESTS . . .

Your breath plays an important role in all oral sex, and particularly with the Air Head. The penis is highly sensitive to temperature changes, and your exhalations will warm up his head and shaft while your inhalations will cool it off again. You may want to try drinking cold water or hot tea before going down on him to see how he responds.

TECHNIQUE

- Lick your lips or use your index finger to paint them with lube as you look into his eyes seductively.
- Wrap your index finger and thumb around the base of his cock.
- Open your wet mouth over his penis and lower it over his head and shaft as you exhale deeply. Don't close your lips over him, but allow incidental contact with your lips, teeth, tongue, and roof of your mouth.
- Once you've lowered your lips as far as you're comfortable going, bring your wide-open mouth back to the tip of his cock as you inhale slowly.

THE GRAND-SLAM BREAKFAST

Sex and food make for a beautiful marriage. Although the Grand-Slam Breakfast doesn't involve any *real* food, it more than makes up for it with direct stimulation of the most nerve-rich area of his penis: the head.

POSITIONING

Kneel on the floor between his knees while he lies in the Swing Set position.

TECHNIQUE

- Begin with the "syrup": Apply lube to his penis by squeezing it out of your clenched fist and letting it drip down his head and shaft.
- Create a "pancake" with your hand: Use a flat, wet palm to rub in circular motions over the head of the penis.
- Replace the pancake with the "juice": Close your soaking wet fingers over the head of his penis and twist as though you're juicing an orange.

VARIATIONS AND ADVANCED TECHNIQUES

Rub the lube all over your breasts and use them to spread "syrup" all over his cock.

DR. JESS SUGGESTS . . .

You can modify most of these techniques by skipping a step or changing the order to your liking in most cases. But you can't skip step number one of the Grand-Slam Breakfast! Without syrup (lube), the pancake (your flat palm) and juice (twisting hand) will be full of friction and leave him in pain. Remember: The wetter the better is the golden rule of all these sizzling tongue and touch techniques.

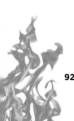

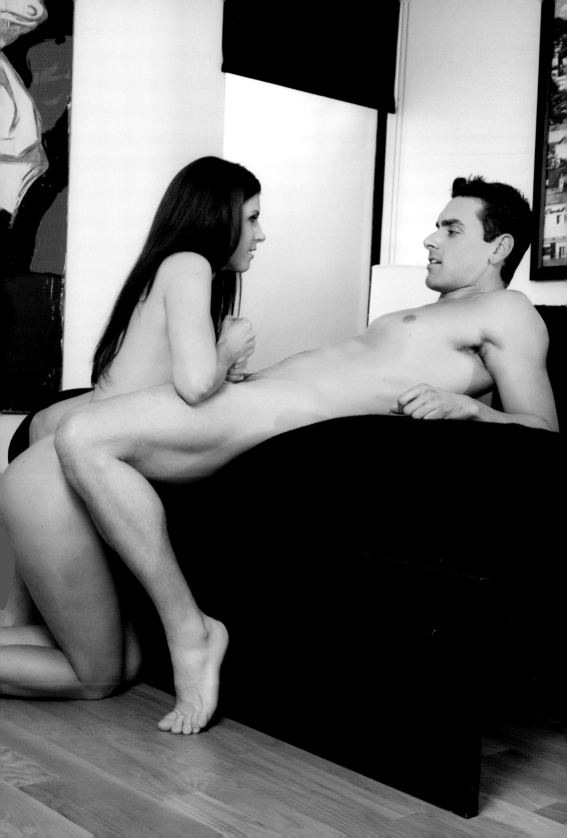

THE TASTE TESTER

The tip of his penis and the frenulum are two of his most sensitive erogenous zones, and the Taste Tester lets you warm him up by playing with both at the same time.

POSITIONING

Position yourself between his legs as he assumes the Gimme More position.

TECHNIQUE

- Apply lots of lube to his penis using your fingers or lips.
- Wrap your fingers around his shaft and place both thumbs on the underside of his penis against his frenulum.
- Use your thumbs to massage small circles against his coronal ridge and frenulum, with your right thumb moving in a clockwise direction and your left thumb moving counterclockwise.
- Suck on the very top of his head and flick his meatus, or pee hole, with your tongue.

VARIATIONS AND ADVANCED TECHNIQUES

If you taste a little precum, stretch it out by pressing your flat tongue against the tip of his penis as you look up at him playfully.

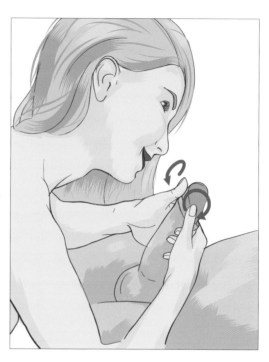

THE LIFESAVER

Play with the Lifesaver to stimulate the highly responsive coronal ridge and make his shaft ache for deeper pleasure.

POSITIONING

Try out the Lifesaver in the Lusty T or the Spread Eagle position.

TECHNIQUE

- Wrap your lips around your teeth to protect his sensitive skin and lower your mouth over his cock until you reach the coronal ridge.
- Twist to the left and right in circular motions.

VARIATIONS AND ADVANCED TECHNIQUES

As you twist, flick your tongue against his frenulum with heavy pressure.

DR. JESS SUGGESTS . . .

If he's uncircumcised, scoop your tongue around inside of his foreskin without retracting it. Use your hands to hold it in place.

THE HIGH FIVE

Use both hands to enjoy his size and cover as much surface area as possible while you stroke his penis.

POSITIONING

High Five him while in the Lusty T or the Reverse Cowgirl.

TECHNIQUE

- Place your lubed, flat palms against the sides of his penis and stroke up and down, allowing your middle fingers to meet at the top.
- Be sure to flex your fingers so that you maintain firm pressure and allow the bones in your palm to press against his hard cock.

VARIATIONS AND ADVANCED TECHNIQUES

If one of your hands is already occupied with some other sexy body part, just use one flat palm to stroke against the underside of his penis as you press it into his abdomen.

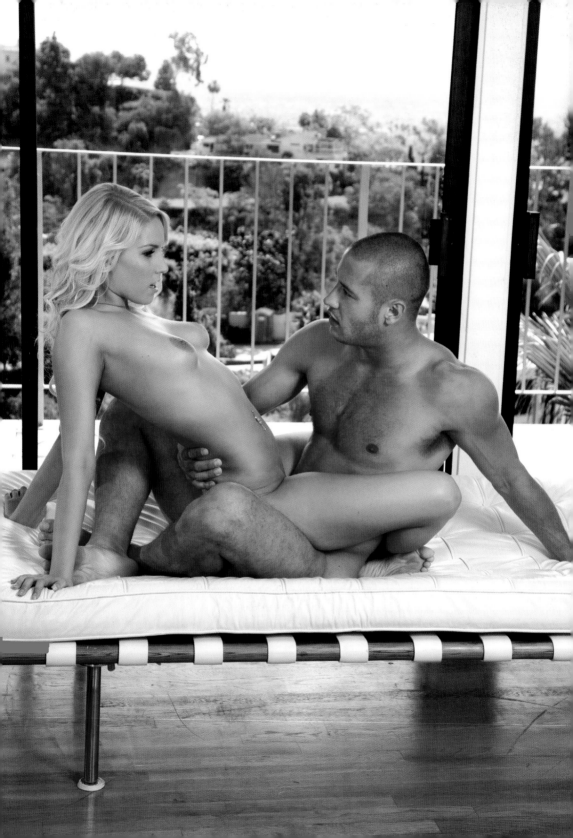

CHAPTER 7

HOTTER TRICKS TO DRIVE HIM WILD

NOW THAT YOU'VE GOT HIS ATTENTION, it's time to turn up the heat and make him quiver with fiery pleasure. Not only will these moves intensify his sexual response, but they will also prime him for an orgasm he won't soon forget.

Although not intended to put him over the edge, don't be surprised if his hips start thrusting and his heavy breathing turns to climactic moaning and uncontrollable gyrations.

If you think he's approaching his point of no return (i.e., he's going to blow his load!) and you're not quite ready (hey, you need to get yours, too, right?), slow your pace, ease up on the pressure, and go back to one of the hot moves from the previous section. On the other hand, if one of these Hotter Tricks to Drive Him Wild seems to push his hottest buttons, tuck it away into your sexual arsenal for your next spontaneous quickie.

THE OTHER WOMAN

It is perfectly normal to be attracted to people other than your partner, and fantasies are a natural extension of this attraction. The Other Woman lets you play with new sensations to mimic the feeling of being touched by a brand-new set of hands.

POSITIONING

Ask your man to assume the Gimme More position and sit behind him so that you can reach around to stroke his cock.

TECHNIQUE

- Get your hand nice and slippery with lube.
- Use a backhand grip beginning in a thumbs-down position to grasp the base of his penis with all five fingers.
- Stroke upward until your thumb and index finger reach the ridge, and then lower your hand all the way back down to the base.

VARIATIONS AND ADVANCED TECHNIQUES

Blindfold him and whisper in his ear to cultivate the fantasy of the Other Woman: "I know lots of women want to get their hands on this big hard cock."

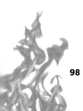

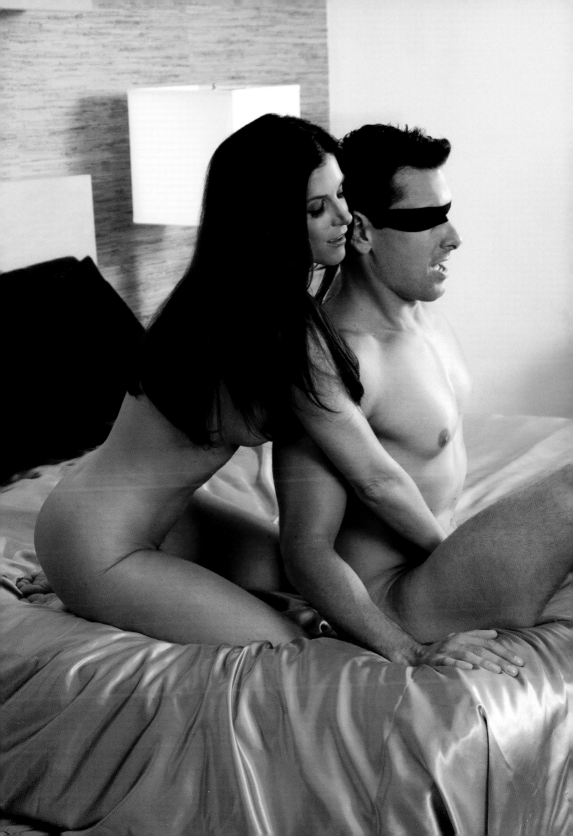

BETTER THAN OKAY

Two is almost always better than one! So use both hands to rub his shaft and sensitive corona to get him going and prepare him for an extraordinary orgasm.

POSITIONING

Try Better Than Okay in the Director's Chair or Spread Eagle position.

TECHNIQUE

- Use your index finger and thumb of each hand to make two okay signs.
- Start with your okay signs at the base of his shaft and work your way up to the coronal ridge, applying enough pressure to let your fingers "pop" over his head.
- Alternate your stroking patterns and twist each okay sign in the opposite direction as you stroke with lots of lube.

VARIATIONS AND ADVANCED TECHNIQUES

Use your two okay signs to stroke the shaft while you suck on the head of his penis with soft, wet lips.

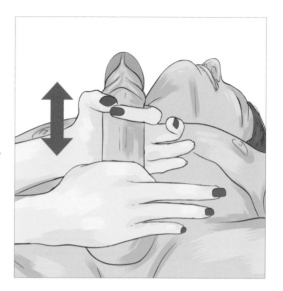

SEXY WRINGER

The Sexy Wringer may remind you of wringing out the laundry, but there's nothing chorelike about making him squirm with pleasure. Be sure to use lots of lube as you work your way from the base to the tip of his penis.

POSITIONING

For the ultimate in pleasure and to ensure you can work from the very base of his member, kneel on the floor (atop a pillow) as he assumes the Swing Set position.

TECHNIQUE

- Slather his cock with lube.
- Wrap both hands around the shaft of his penis, one above the other.
- Twist to the right with one hand as you simultaneously twist to the left with the other hand, as though you're wringing out a wet shirt—but not with the same intensity.
- Once this motion has become fluid, continue your wringing as you move up the shaft to grasp his head with your upper hand. As you move your hands up and down his hard cock, keep the pace smooth and slow like the gradual climb of an elevator.

VARIATIONS AND ADVANCED TECHNIQUES

Once your upper hand reaches the coronal ridge, squeeze and release with your thumb and middle finger to create a pulsing sensation.

VARIATION: THE TWISTER

The Twister is a variation of the Sexy Wringer, but instead of twisting your hands in opposite directions, use your mouth and one hand to turn away from one another.

RINGMASTER

Catapult your standard blow job to new heights with the addition of simple hand seals that trap the blood in the penis to keep it hard and make it tingle with excitement.

POSITIONING

The Ringmaster works in almost all positions as long as your hands are free to reach down between his legs.

TECHNIQUE

- Wrap your thumb and index finger around the base of his shaft and press down against his pelvis.
- Maintain this grip while you lick, blow, kiss, and suck away.
- If he's circumcised, retract his foreskin and ask him how far he likes you to pull it down before getting started.

VARIATIONS AND ADVANCED TECHNIQUES

- Wrap your thumbs around the back of his balls and curl your index fingers around the base of his penis, allowing them meet between his shaft and abdomen.
- You should create a full closed circle with your fingers and thumb and can adjust the ring to fit snugly as you suck on his balls, shaft, and head.

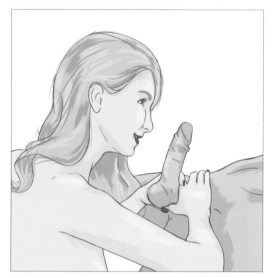

DR. JESS SUGGESTS . . .

Cock rings are one of the most common sex toys for men. They are used to trap blood in the penis, keeping it harder for longer and heightening orgasmic response. The classic cock ring wraps around the base of the penis while the adjustable ones extend around both the base of the penis and the scrotum. The Ringmaster is a human cock ring that's even hotter than its rubber, metal, and leather counterparts because it involves more skin-to-skin contact.

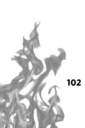

THE BALL GAME

The scrotal sac is very sensitive to the touch, and it's no surprise given that they contain the testes, which are a hotbed of male hormone production. So when you're heading down between his legs, don't neglect the male sex glands—the payoff can be huge!

POSITIONING

Play the Ball Game while your partner lies on his back in the Gimme More position or stands erect in the Stand at Attention position. Better yet, lie on your back and ask him to Sit on My Face.

TECHNIQUE

- Press your palm against the back of his balls while you shove them in your own face and draw a big slow W over the front side.

- Pucker your moist lips and gently suck only on the skin of his scrotal sac.
- Gently suck a whole ball into your mouth and twirl your tongue around it.
- Use the pointy tip of your tongue to draw a figure eight around both balls.
- Cup his balls with one warm hand and slowly pull them downward as you suck upward on his cock from base to tip.
- Slather lube all over his balls and rub your face in them as you exhale deeply.

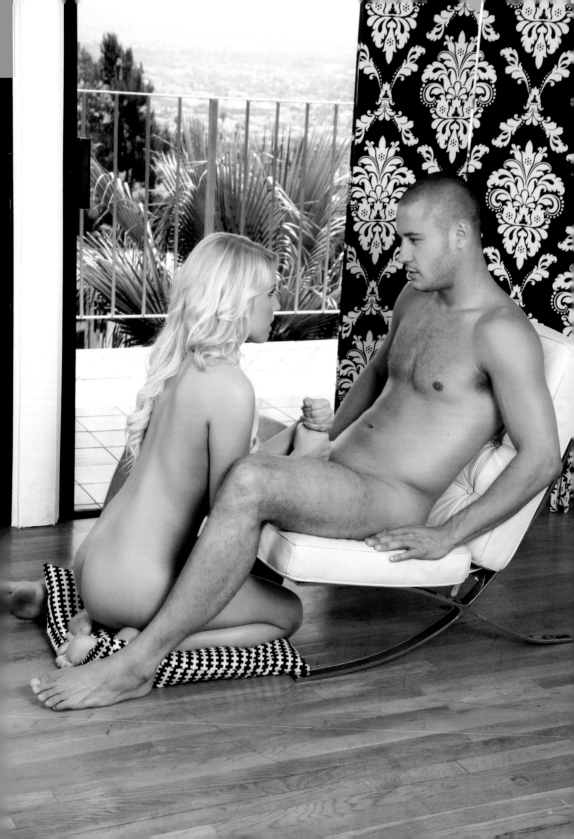

MILK WOMAN

While every man enjoys the thrill of a standard up-and-down-stroke hand job (as long as there is sufficient lubrication), changing up the direction of your strokes can activate new sexual responses and trigger activity in various parts of the sexual brain.

POSITIONING

You can play with the Milk Woman in multiple positions, including Director's Chair, Swing Set, Gimme More, and Stand at Attention.

TECHNIQUE

- Grasp the base of his penis with your lubed right hand so that your thumb and index finger are pressed against his abdomen.
- Squeeze tightly and pull his penis toward you, allowing your hand to pop off of the tip.
- As your right hand approaches his head, add your left hand at the base and pull up, alternating hands as though you're milking the cum right out of him.
- Use firm pressure and make sure that your stroking is constant.

VARIATIONS AND ADVANCED TECHNIQUES

- Try the Milk Woman while kneeling behind your man as he gets into the Stand at Attention position. Poke your head between his legs to lick and suck his perineum, bum, or balls while you reach around his sides to milk his penis.

THE FLICKER

Enhance your basic sucking blow job by stimulating three of his hottest spots with your sexy tongue.

POSITIONING

You'll need to get down between his legs to flick his hot spots, so try one of these positions: Gimme More, Lie Back and Take It, Director's Chair, or Sit on My Face.

TECHNIQUE

- Suck away until he's hard and throbbing, and then use your tongue to flick his meatus (pee hole).
- Continue sucking and use a flat tongue to create friction against his frenulum. Alternate between a wide, flat tongue and the pointy tip as you stimulate this scream-worthy spot on the underside of his penis.
- As he gets more worked up, lower your lips all the way to the bottom third of his shaft and flick your tongue against his base. If possible, flick it up and down and back and forth to activate different nerve endings.

VARIATIONS AND ADVANCED TECHNIQUES

Try the Flicker in the Giraffe position to elongate your mouth. If you can take his penis deep enough, use your tongue to flick all around the base against his pubic mound.

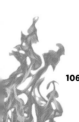

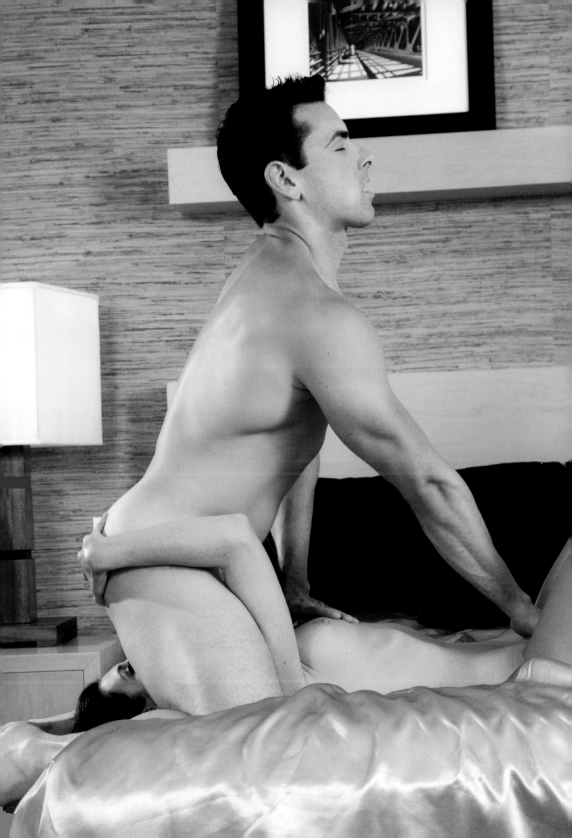

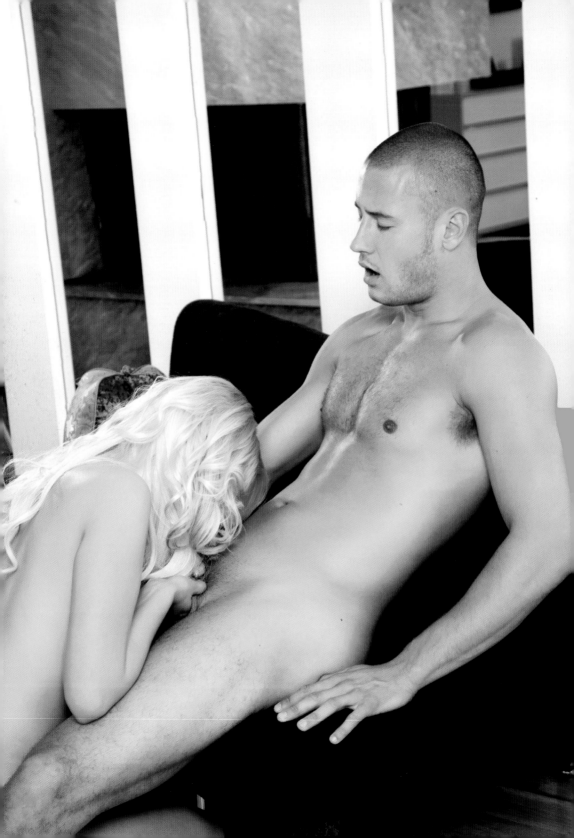

AROUND THE WORLD

Balls and shaft and head—oh my! He can have it all and so can you with the Around the World technique.

POSITIONING

The Around the World works well with your man in the Stand at Attention position as you sit on the edge of the bed in front of him.

TECHNIQUE

- Look into his eyes and tell him that you're craving his hot juices.
- Play with his balls with one hand and use the other to grip the lower half of his shaft.
- Wrap your tongue all around his head and coronal ridge, twisting back and forth and moaning with pleasure.
- Tell him how good he feels inside of your mouth!

VARIATIONS AND ADVANCED TECHNIQUES

Slide your lips halfway down his shaft and wrap your tongue all the way around. Work your way up to the tip gradually as you continue wrapping your tongue in full circles.

DR. JESS SUGGESTS . . .

Be a tease! Use Around the World to take a break from sucking as you loop your tongue all around his cock without taking it into your mouth. Let him beg for it while you look into his eyes with a devilish smile. Ask him to tell you just *how badly* he wants it as you continue to twirl to your heart's content.

THE CHERRY POP

This technique not only feels good, but also the natural sounds of sex enhance the mood for you and your lover.

POSITIONING

Straddle your man in the Reverse Cowgirl position as you perform the Cherry Pop.

TECHNIQUE

- Use lots of lube as you rub his shaft between your flat palms as though you're starting a fire.
- Breathe all over the head of his cock to tease him a little.
- Ask him if he wants to put it in your mouth. (It's obviously a rhetorical question!)
- Slowly lower your lips over his cock until you pass over the coronal ridge.
- Suck gently below the coronal ridge with very little movement. This should be a tiny suck in which your lips don't slide more than ¼ to ½ inch (6mm to 1.3 cm) up or down.
- Keep rubbing his shaft with your wet palms while you pop your lips off the tip, making a sexy (and possible sloppy) popping sound. Pop a few more times before alternating your pops with your tiny sucks below the corona.

VARIATIONS AND ADVANCED TECHNIQUES

As you pop your lips off the head of his penis, curl your tongue around his head to create more suction.

DR. JESS SUGGESTS . . .

From silent to thundering and everything in between, sex sounds are a natural part of the erotic experience, so try not to hold back. When we stifle our moans, alter our primal grunts, and hold our breath, we also restrain our sexual response. Don't be afraid to make noises (slurps, gulps, pops, hisses, groans, whistles, etc.) during sex play, because they're all part of your authentic encounter.

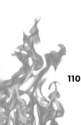

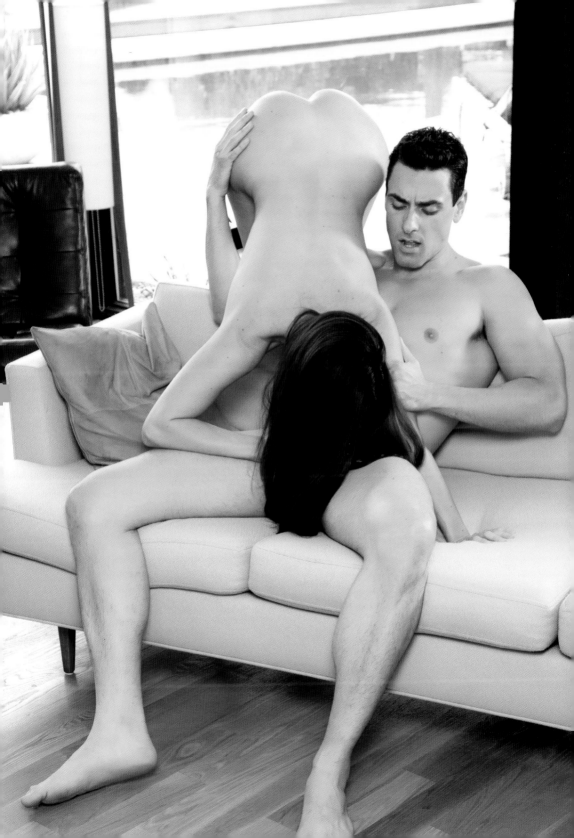

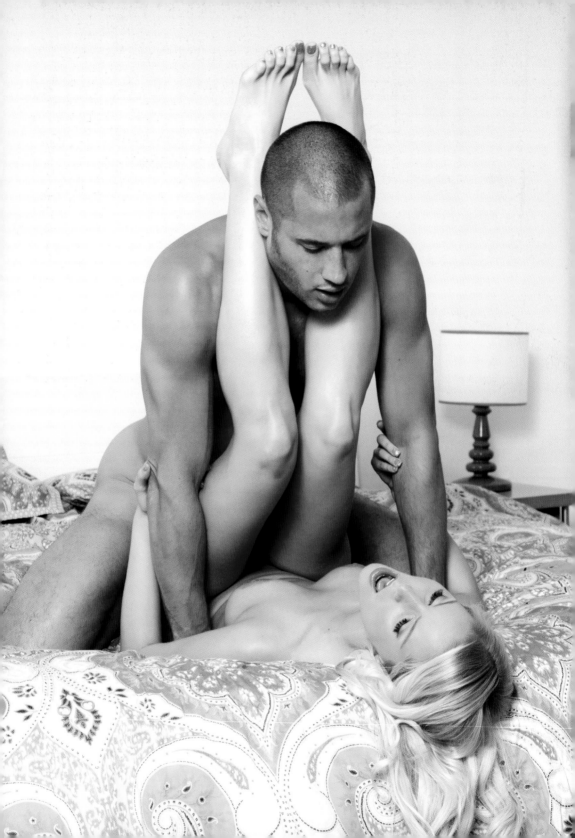

CHAPTER 8

THE HOTTEST TECHNIQUES FOR MIND-BLOWING ORGASMS

ONCE YOU'VE WORKED HIM UP INTO AN UNSTOPPABLE SEXUAL FRENZY, it's time to pull out the big guns and finish him off with one (or two) of your hottest techniques. Whether you like to use your hands, your mouth, or both, you're sure to keep him coming back for more.

And as hot as these physical techniques may be for him, the more *you* are into it, the more you'll both get out of it. So find a way to make sure you're feeling hot and heavy, too:

- Rub yourself against his legs or a pillow.
- Grab his fingers and show him how to use them.
- Fantasize about something naughty or nice.
- Encourage him to tease you with a little dirty talk.
- Breathe deeply and release whatever sounds come naturally—don't worry if you don't sound like a lady or a porn star, because when it comes to sex, you're really just a horny animal!

MASSAGE-PARLOR TWIST

This is a go-to move for hand-job enthusiasts. Just a handful of strokes will have him melting like putty in your hand.

POSITIONING

Lie or kneel next to him in the Lusty T or kneel between his legs as he assumes the Swing Set position.

TECHNIQUE

- Cover his cock in lube.
- Begin with a forehand grip around the base of his shaft.
- Stroke upward and twist counterclockwise when you reach the head of his cock.
- Turn back clockwise as you run your grip back down the shaft to the base.

VARIATIONS AND ADVANCED TECHNIQUES

Alternate between your left and right hands or use a spare hand to massage his balls.

TONGUE VIBRATOR ▶

Vibrators aren't just for frisky women! Many men also love the sensation of pulsations on their tender spots. In fact, some men say that a vibrating cock ring can catapult their sexual response into new dimensions.

POSITIONING

Anything goes as long as you're giving him a blow job!

TECHNIQUE

- Make a buzzing sound as you suck up and down his shaft or kiss all around his balls.
- If buzzing feels unnatural, try some exaggerated moaning to create reverberations against his smooth skin.

VARIATIONS AND ADVANCED TECHNIQUES

Buy a stretchy vibrating cock ring and slide it onto your tongue before going down on him.

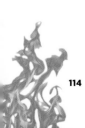

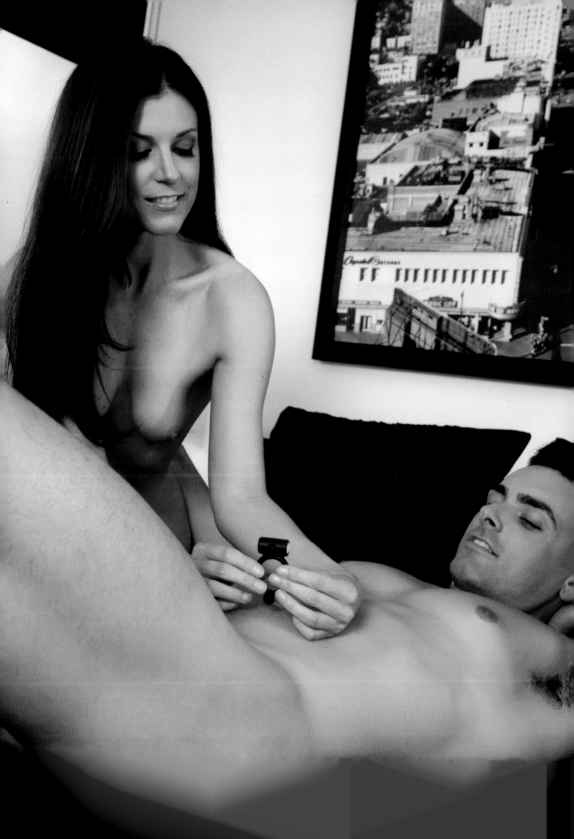

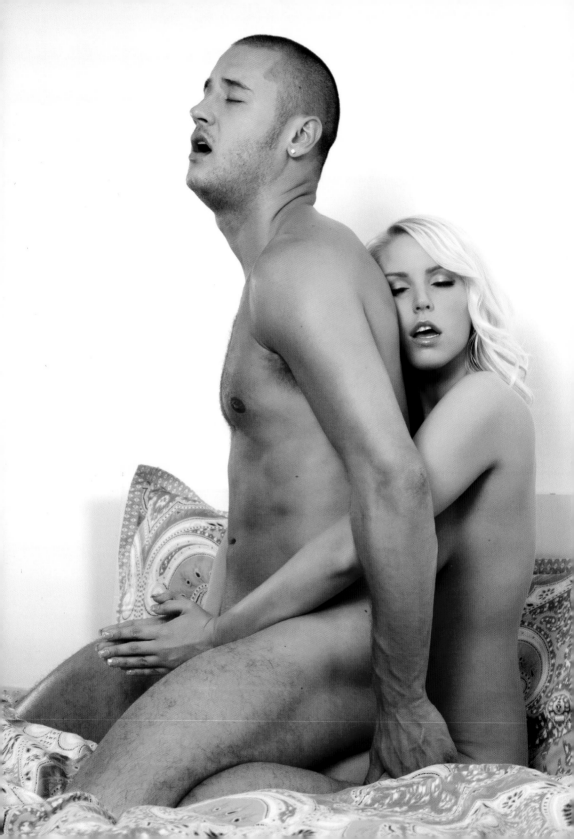

LIKE A PRAYER

Have him singing your praises as you take him to new heights with the Like a Prayer technique.

POSITIONING

Have your man sit in the Gimme More position and cozy up behind him, reaching your hands around to touch his cock.

TECHNIQUE

- Rub some lube between your palms to warm them up and place your hands in prayer position.
- Once he's hard, lower your hands over his cock, beginning with the base of your palms and keeping your fingertips pointing up toward his head.
- Once you reach the base, open up your index and middle fingers before moving back to the tip and returning your hands to prayer position.
- Apply firm pressure as you stroke your hands up and down in prayer position.

VARIATIONS AND ADVANCED TECHNIQUES

Try the Like a Prayer with your man in the Lie Back and Take It position, kneeling between his legs. As your hands work their way down his throbbing shaft, suck the tip of his cock with pursed lips.

COCK AND LOAD

If he loves a tight grip *and* has a sensitive frenulum, he's sure to love the Cock and Load.

POSITIONING

Kneel between his legs while he assumes the Lie Back and Take It or Gimme More position.

TECHNIQUE

- Work him into a desperate frenzy before getting started with this technique.
- Wrap both hands around the base of his lubed cock, interlacing your fingers on the upper side of it.
- Point both thumbs upward toward his tip against the underside of his penis.
- Squeeze and stroke upward and trace small circles or hearts with your thumbs as they pass over his frenulum.
- Maintain a tight, wet grip as you rub him up and down at a rhythmic pace.

VARIATIONS AND ADVANCED TECHNIQUES

Pulse your thumbs against his frenulum to create an electric charge of orgasmic energy with each stroke.

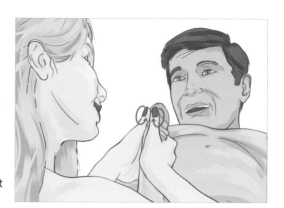

MORE TO LOVE

This is a sure-fire way to finish him off and leave him aching for more of you, you, YOU! Using two hands allows you to grip him tightly and mimic the sensations of hot sex using your palms and all ten fingers.

POSITIONING

This move is very versatile! You can try the More to Love in the Director's Chair, Swing Set, Lie Back and Take It, and Gimme More positions.

TECHNIQUE

- Rub a generous amount of lube between your hands to get them nice and warm.
- Wrap both hands around the base of his penis, interlacing your fingers.
- Slip and slide from the base to tip using firm pressure and a steady pace.
- As you approach the head, twist your hands around the coronal ridge in a fluid motion.

VARIATIONS AND ADVANCED TECHNIQUES

If he likes a little extra pressure, pulse with an extra squeeze with each stroke at the very base of his cock.

DR. JESS SUGGESTS . . .

Pulsing sensations can bring on super-intense orgasms, because they mimic the contractions experienced right before and during orgasm. Some men even like it if you pulse gently as they come to heighten their sexual response.

THE TWIST AND SHOUT ▶

A different take on the Massage-Parlor Twist, this technique is totally moan-worthy because you'll be pleasuring from base to tip.

POSITIONING

Try the Twist and Shout in the Lusty T or the Reverse Cowgirl.

TECHNIQUE

- Apply lots of lube to your dominant hand.
- Begin with the Other Woman grip, with your right palm facing away from you and your thumb pointing down. (See page 98.)
- Firmly grasp the shaft at the base and slide up toward the head; your palm should still face away from you.
- When you reach the head, twist your hand clockwise around the head and over the top so that your palm ends facing you and you're still gripping the penis from the far side. Pay attention to the ridge and frenulum as you perform the twist, because these areas can be highly sensitive.
- Slide down the other side of the penis and repeat!

VARIATIONS AND ADVANCED TECHNIQUES

Once you're comfortable with this move and it becomes one fluid movement, alternate between your right and left hands as you twist and he shouts!

TWISTED SISTER

The Twisted Sister is the oral version of the manual Twist and Shout. It's a great finishing move to make his head spin with pleasure.

POSITIONING

You'll need to kneel or lie at his side in the Lusty T position to play with the Twisted Sister.

TECHNIQUE

- Begin at his side so that you are facing the profile of his penis.
- Wrap your lips around his penis so that your top and bottom lips contact the sides of his penis; if he looks down at you, he should see your face in profile.
- Lower your tightened lips down the shaft of his penis.
- When you reach the base, suck upward toward the head and keep your tongue pressed flat against his shaft.
- Before your reach the ridge of the penis, make a quarter turn so that you now face his abdomen and can look him in the eye; maintain the suction during this fluid twisting movement.
- As you make the quarter turn, wrap your slobbery tongue around the frenulum and corona.
- You may want to practice this one on a cucumber or dildo first.

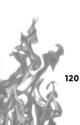

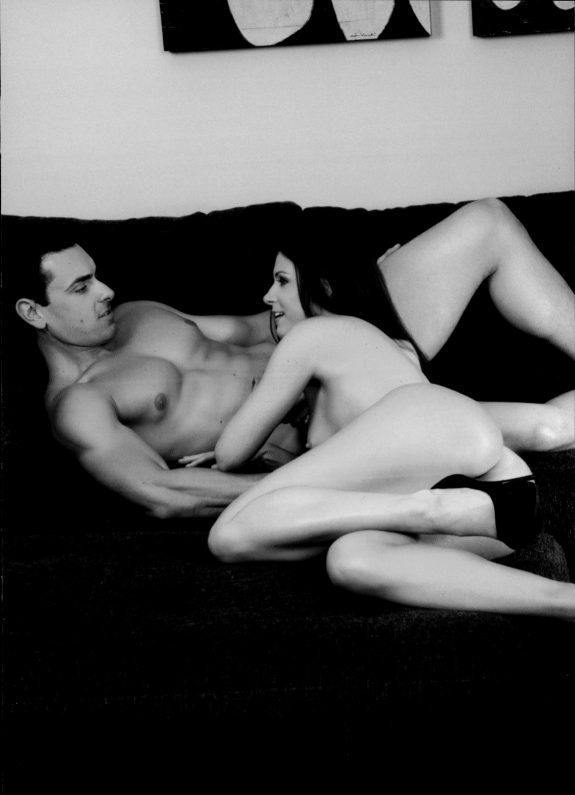

THE PENIS GURU

This technique is sure to become a go-to move as you stroke the *entire* penis, including the inner bulb that is so often neglected.

POSITIONING

Kneel between his legs in the Stand at Attention or Director's Chair position.

TECHNIQUE

- Lube up both hands and place three fingers against the back of his perineum (near his butt hole).
- Use the other hand to create a seal at the base of his penis with your thumb and index finger.
- Slide your wet lips down his shaft toward the base.
- Suck upward as you glide your three fingers forward along his perineum.
- Be sure you're stroking forward along the perineum (toward the front of his body) as you suck upward, and then stroke backward as you lower your lips down his shaft. This will ensure that your stroke really covers the whole delicious cock from inner base to tip.

VARIATIONS AND ADVANCED TECHNIQUES

Create a tunnel with your hand and soak it in lube. Attach this tunnel to your mouth to create the sensation that you're sucking deeper toward his base.

DR. JESS SUGGESTS . . .

MRI images of penile-vaginal intercourse show that the penis is boomerang-shaped with the base bending back against the perineum inside the body. As you stroke the perineum, you're rubbing the deepest portion of his inner penis.

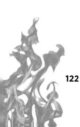

I CAN'T BELIEVE IT'S NOT VAGINA

Believe it or not, your hands alone can make his toes curl and make you the center of his every sexual daydream and fantasy—you just need a lot of warmth, lube, and the I Can't Believe It's Not Vagina technique. Blindfold him, work him up by caressing his entire body, and see if he can tell the difference!

POSITIONING

You can use this technique in the Reverse Cowgirl or Spread Eagle position.

TECHNIQUE

- Place a flat, lubed palm against the base of his shaft with your fingers facing upward toward the head.
- Place your other lube-soaked hand at a 90-degree angle with your fingers facing toward the side.
- Apply firm pressure to create suction as you slide upward to the head and back down to the base.
- As you approach the base, go deeper by allowing your second hand to turn outward without relieving any of the pressure and suction.

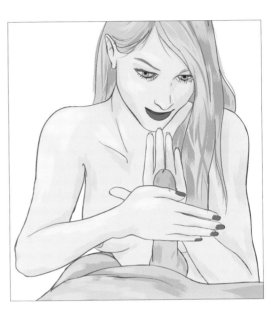

THE MONEY MOVE

Make him moan with blazing-hot passion and leave him dreaming of your magic lips with one of the tightest blow-job grips: the Money Move.

POSITIONING

Kneel between his legs as he assumes the Lie Back and Take It or Gimme More position.

TECHNIQUE

- Use your tongue to cover your lower teeth and your upper lip to cover your upper teeth.
- Rub some lube on your upper lip and slide your lips over his shaft, pressing your tongue firmly against the underside of his hard cock.
- Make whatever noises (sucking, slurping, moaning) that come naturally to you and try to maintain strong suction as you taste his throbbing manhood with your lips and tongue. Use your covered teeth to grip him with firm pressure.
- Work him over at a fairly quick pace, maintaining a steady rhythm until he comes.

DR. JESS SUGGESTS . . .

Although you need to cover your lower teeth with your tongue for the Money Move, don't stick your tongue too far out, because this can make it difficult to take him more deeply into your mouth. Just stick your tongue out enough to be sure that your teeth don't make any contact with his cock. And remember that a tasty, flavored lube is absolutely necessary because your upper lip won't lubricate on its own.

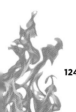

THE HALF AND HALF

Want the best of both worlds? Use the strength of your hands to grip his lower shaft while your lips slide all around his sensitive head.

POSITIONING

Try the Half and Half with your man in the Director's Chair position.

TECHNIQUE

- Wrap your wet hands around his base in the More to Love grip (page 119). Slide sensuously up and down the lower half with firm pressure.
- Suck on the upper half with the Money Move (page 124), covering your teeth with your tongue and upper lips.

VARIATIONS AND ADVANCED TECHNIQUES

- Pulse with your hand at the base and your lips and tongue at the coronal ridge simultaneously.
- Add a twist at the head and slurp away!

DR. JESS SUGGESTS . . .

Change up your positioning at each encounter to produce new reactions and sensations. It's amazing how much a change of angle can do to enhance the way his body responds to your erotic touch.

THE PROFESSIONAL

While the head of the penis might be the most sensitive in terms of innervation, the bottom third is often the hot spot for orgasmic response. If you want to make him come with speed and intensity, wrap your lips and tongue around this sensitive area and suck away.

POSITIONING

You'll need to get deeper for this move, so try it in the Giraffe position with your man standing next to the bed.

TECHNIQUE

- Lie back and grasp the base of his penis with an okay sign so that you can control the depth of penetration.
- Pull him into your mouth and suck on the lower third of the shaft with firm pressure. Stick your tongue out a little and use both your lips and your tongue to inhale him deeply into your mouth with lots of pressure and suction.
- Keep the pace steady and let his thrusting determine the pace.

- If you can't go as deep as you'd like to, use one lubed hand as an extension of your mouth: Wrap your wet hand around his head and slide it down, lowering your lips right after it in one fluid motion until your hand reaches the base.

DR. JESS SUGGESTS . . .
Cup his balls while you're sucking on his cock. As he approaches orgasm, you'll feel them tighten and lift up toward his body.

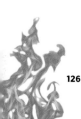

To Swallow or Not to Swallow?

It's really not much of a question. If you're into it, then soak it all in—and if you're not, simply move on. There is an infinite number of alternatives to swallowing, and you really should only engage in sexual behaviors that make you feel great—physically and emotionally.

IF YOU'RE INTERESTED IN SWALLOWING, CONSIDER THESE OPTIONS:

• Take him deep into your throat and let him come as you exaggerate your gulping sounds and gaze seductively into his eyes.

• Suck only on his swollen head as he comes so that you can control how much cum you swallow at once.

• Open your mouth wide and stroke his shaft as he releases his hot cum all over your tongue.

• Tell him how good he tastes.

• Use a flavored lube to enhance the taste or wash it down with your favorite beverage.

• Ease up your pressure while he's coming and sensually wrap your wide, flat tongue around the underside of his penis.

IF SWALLOWING JUST ISN'T YOUR THING, YOU HAVE LOTS OF OPTIONS AS LONG AS HE GIVES YOU NOTICE BEFORE HE'S ABOUT TO EJACULATE:

• Ask him to spray his hot load onto your chest: "I want it all over my tits!"

• Suck on his throbbing head as he comes, but discreetly spit it into a mug of water or a towel instead of swallowing.

• Beg him to come in your mouth and let it drip out into a big sticky mess instead of swallowing.

• Use your hands to engulf his warm cum.

• Use a flavored condom for oral sex!

• Bring him to the point of no return and then hop on his hard cock to let him come inside of your pussy.

DR. JESS SUGGESTS . . .

If your lover likes the sensation of swallowing, try throat Kegels while you're sucking him off: Lower your lips halfway down his shaft (or deeper if you're comfortable) and swallow deeply, exaggerating the sound and gulping sensation to wrap your entire lips around his shaft with suction and pressure.

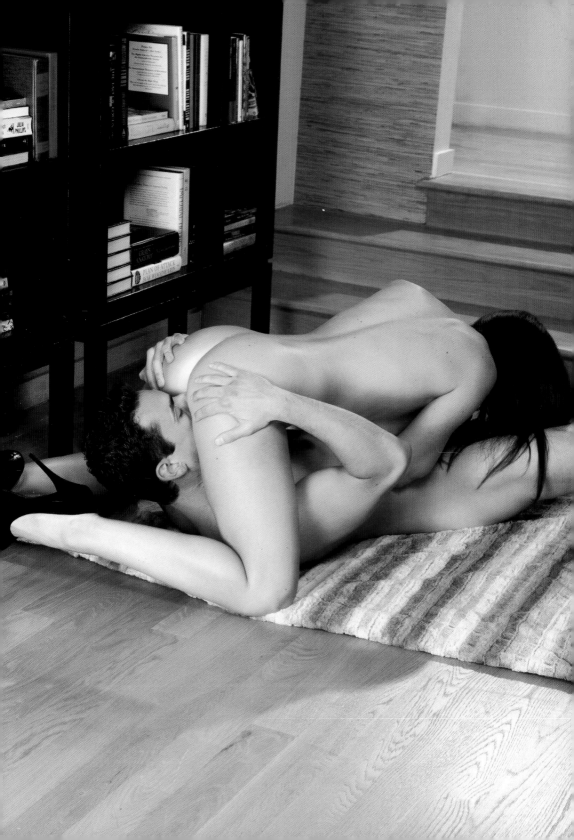

CHAPTER 9

SEX PLAY FOR TWO

NOW THAT YOU'VE MASTERED A WHOLE NEW SET OF TECHNIQUES, it's time to put them together and experiment until they become a part of your natural repertoire. The last thing you want to be thinking of when you're getting it on and getting yourselves off is the technical aspect of your sex play. So sit back, relax, and let your lips, fingers, and tongues do all the work while your mind wanders into the depths of your hedonistic desire.

Advanced techniques can help you turn up the heat, but they're only one component of sexual satisfaction. Keeping things fresh, experimenting with new approaches, and developing meaningful connections are also key to steamy sex. So if you're looking to up the ante, read on to check out some of the ways to promote mutual pleasure and multiple orgasms while exploring new territory with your sexy lover.

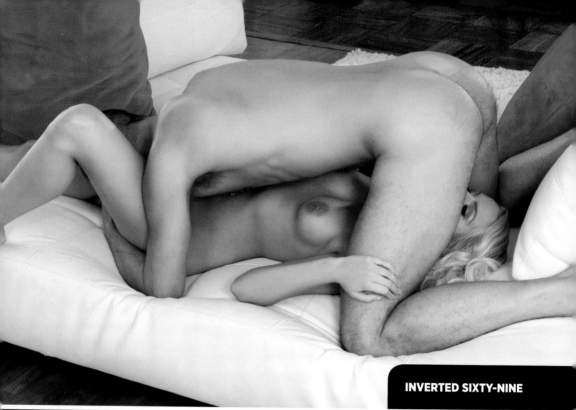

INVERTED SIXTY-NINE

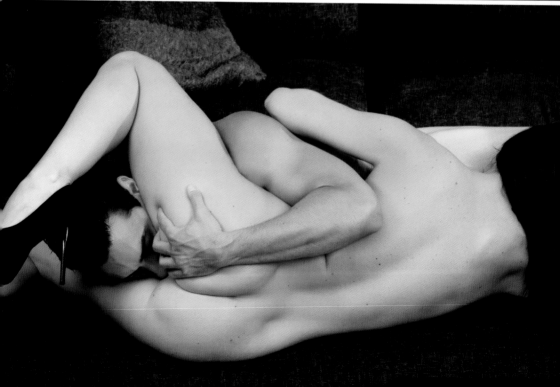

SIDE BY SIDE

SHARING IS CARING: 69 AND OTHER VARIATIONS

What's better than oral sex? Oral sex for two!

It may be polite to take turns, but hot sex often precludes good manners. After all, tearing off clothes and shoving your tongue in all places imaginable don't exactly amount to the pinnacle of politeness—so why stop there? Instead of taking turns, make every moment count and be greedy! All these exciting tips, tricks, and licks can be adapted to make sure that you both experience optimal pleasure simultaneously. Sure, giving may be fun, and many great lovers get off on seeing their partners aroused. But there is something especially erotic about synchronous oral sex—it's as though two-become-one in the most intimate of ways.

You've probably heard of the 69 position, but once you start bending, flexing, and twisting, the possibilities for dual indulgence are endless! Play with these variations of the traditional 69 to experience mutual pleasure and maybe even simultaneous orgasms.

TRADITIONAL *SOIXANTE-NEUF*

Everything just sounds hotter in French, doesn't it? In the traditional 69 position, the man lies on his back and the woman gets on her knees over his face, so that he can muff dive to his heart's content. She bends over to dive in on the action, stroking, sucking, licking, and blowing his cock simultaneously.

INVERTED SIXTY-NINE

In this position, the woman lies back while the man kneels over her face (facing down toward her feet) at an angle that allows her to suck his cock into her eager mouth. He bends down and licks, kisses, and moans away at her pussy.

SIDE BY SIDE

This is the politically correct version of the 69 position because neither the man nor the woman assumes the superior position. Kidding! This is a great position for dual gratification, because it's easy on the back and allows you to dive deep into those sexy nether regions. Both partners lie on their sides facing one another with their heads on opposite sides of the bed and their hands free to reach around and explore their partner's backside.

ON THE EDGE OF YOUR SEAT

This position may require a bit of practice, but once you get the hang of it, you'll be happy you took the time. Begin in the traditional 69 position, with his legs hanging off the bed as in the Swing Set position. Once you're comfortable, he sits up and she supports herself in an assisted handstand position or by wrapping her arms around his hips as the sucking and blowing continue without interruption.

WHY NOT?

This marvelous position requires some flexibility, but it is a rewarding payoff for all those morning yoga sessions. The man sits flat on the ground or bed with his legs spread and the woman stands with her legs on the outside of his legs facing toward his feet. She bends over and places her hands on the floor or mattress for support and bends her knees as much as is needed to be comfortable and be able to suck on his cock. Her butt is in his face and he gets a great view as well as the opportunity to plunge his face between her legs from behind.

THE 68

Although only one partner receives oral stimulation in this position, the physical closeness ensures that pleasure will be shared between the two. Just like the traditional 69 position, one partner lies on his or her back while the other lies on top with his or her head at the opposite end. However, the top partner flips onto his or her back to relax while the bottom partner gains full access to the other person's sexiest regions.

MULTIPLE (SUCCESSIVE) ORGASMS FOR WOMEN

If you or your partner enjoys multiple orgasms or wants to explore the possibility of being multiorgasmic, that's great news! However, bear in mind that orgasms (multiple or single) are not sideshow tricks—they're personal, subjective experiences. So if you put pressure on yourself or your partner to perform, you'll take all the fun out of the experience.

As always, do what feels good for you and try these strategies on your own before bringing them into partnered play. Sometimes it's healthy to be selfish! You're more likely to enjoy and learn from the authentic sexual experience without the pressure of worrying about your partner's needs.

Try these approaches to experimenting with multiples.

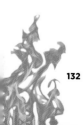

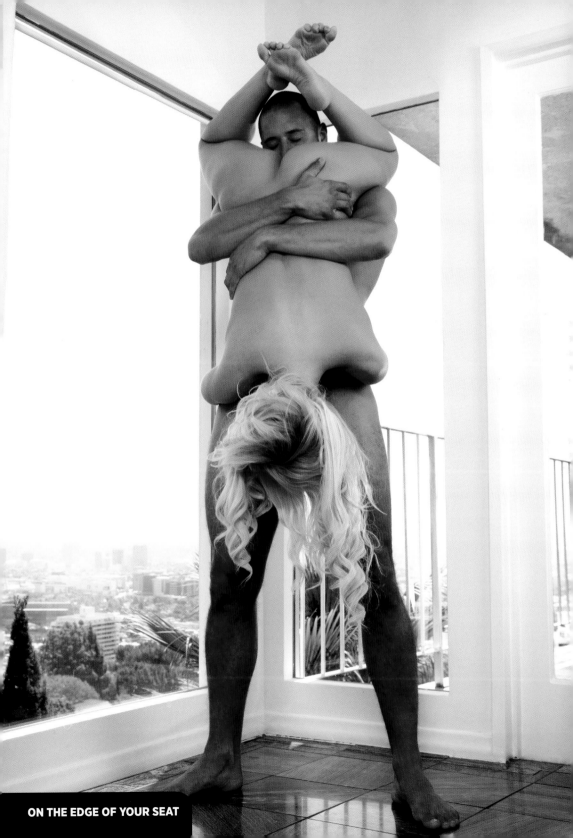

ON THE EDGE OF YOUR SEAT

FULL-BODY WORK-UP

We all have a tendency to pay a ton of attention to the breasts, bum, and genitals while ignoring the rest of the corporeal wonderland during sex. Although there is nothing wrong with focusing on the common erogenous zones, slow and simultaneous stimulation of several body parts at once can heighten orgasmic response, promote full-body orgasms, and bring on more orgasms in one steamy session. Try using a blindfold and caressing the whole body from head to toe, teasing around the vulva and breasts to build up the tension. Later on, when orgasm is imminent, use a spare hand, mouth, toy, pillow, or even toe to touch as much of the body as possible to extend the orgasmic experience.

PLAY WITH FANTASY

Many women (and men) report that their most memorable orgasms begin and end with a hot fantasy. So embrace this! Fantasies that involve people other than your partner in no way constitute cheating—nor are they a reflection of your *real* desires. They are simply fragments of your wildest sexual imagination that come together to create a perfect scenario in your mind for the narrow purpose of getting you off. In one case study of a woman who had more than a hundred orgasms in one sitting, fantasy was identified as essential to meeting her needs, so even if you're not on the path to one hundred orgasms (who has that kind of time?), playing with fantasy is definitely worth exploring.

TEASE IT OUT! AVOID HER HOT SPOTS

Find out where she loves to be touched and which buttons take her to the orgasmic edge. Then use your breath, lips, tongue, and slippery fingers to tease all around these sex zones without actually touching the areas that burn with the most fiery desire. Let them ache for a stroke, kiss, or suck until they can no longer handle it, and then dive in for the win!

PULSE!

Many women enjoy bigger, better, and more orgasms by pulsing on the hood of the clitoris with a finger in between orgasmic contractions. She will have to learn to recognize these contractions to try this technique, but once she does, it's actually quite simple and she can use her hand to guide yours. As soon her PC muscles contract, press firmly for approximately half a second and release following the rhythm of her body's involuntary contractions. Alternatively, you can place your hand over her entire vulva using the Pussy Pocket technique and pulse away (page 30)!

PC SQUEEZES

If the clitoral hood is too sensitive for direct contact, some women can prolong orgasms by purposely contracting and releasing their PC muscle while they're coming. Exercising this muscle regularly is also a must, because it can improve circulation, continence, and sexual response.

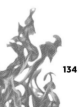

DON'T STOP!

Orgasms rock, but they're not the be-all, end-all of sex, so why stop as soon as you come? Keep going during the afterglow with kisses, hugs, thrusts, snuggles, strokes, licks, and flirtation to carry you through to the next level of sexual excitement.

USE VIBRATORS

More than half of the adult population admits to having used vibrators for sex play, and it's no surprise, because their powerful sensations provide the prolonged, intense stimulation enjoyed by both men and women. In addition the latest research shows that women who use vibrators report higher levels of arousal, lubrication, orgasm, and sexual fulfillment.

TAKE A STEP BACK FROM THE EDGE

Sometimes a quickie is just what the doctor ordered, as it satiates your every desire and leaves you with enough time to catch a few hours of much-needed rest before starting all over again in the morning. But sometimes, sex needs to be drawn out in order to realize it's full potential. That's where a bit of edge play comes in!

Play with your favorite moves to bring her right to the edge of orgasm . . . and then reel her back in without taking her over the top. Do it again and again to make the first (and second and third) orgasm well worth the wait. All the pent-up tension can make her orgasms explosive and sequential. This takes a lot of communication when playing as a pair, so it's best if she tries it out on her own first while masturbating to learn to recognize her point of no return that precedes orgasm.

In fact, although each of these approaches is described for partnered sex, they may be best explored for the first time while masturbating to become familiar with your own unique sexual response.

DR. JESS SUGGESTS . . .

If you try all of these strategies and still don't experience more than one orgasm, that's perfectly okay. The journey is often the hottest part, so enjoy the exploration and rest assured that sex researchers have found that overall sexual satisfaction is not overwhelmingly impacted by the presence or absence of multiples.

ANAL PLAY

The butt is a sensitive, highly innervated area that is associated with both the heights of pleasure and the depths of unnecessarily shameful discharge. The good news for those who enjoy anal sex play is that experts report that very little (if any) feces are actually stored in the rectum. Hooray!

Some people love the idea of butt play while others are totally turned off by it. Whatever your fancy, you definitely fall within the range of "normal"—not that it should matter. Anal sex of all kinds can be pleasurable regardless of your sexual orientation, and some basic hygiene and reeducation may just make for some of the more powerful sexual experiences you can imagine.

Be sure to check out all the fun parts in the rear:

The cheeks: These are the round mounds of gluteal muscles layered with luscious fat.

The crack: This sexy and sensitive space lies between the cheeks; it is great for toying with to build anticipation and some erotic teasing.

The butt hole/anus: The external opening of the anus is usually darker in color and is covered with some hair growth.

Internal sphincter: This valve is located at the lower edge and is controlled by the autonomous (subconscious) nervous system. During comfortable insertion (and expulsion), this sphincter can relax due to rectal flex, which makes accommodating an object more comfortable.

External sphincter: This strong muscle can be tightened and released at will, because it is controlled by the spinal nerve. You can feel your external sphincter by inserting a lubed finger into your anus and practicing contractions of the sphincter muscle—you'll feel your butt squeeze around your finger.

DR. JESS SUGGESTS . . .

The legs of the clitoris can be stimulated through the anus in women, and some women (just like men) can enjoy orgasm through butt play. What does this mean? Both men *and* women can derive intense pleasure through the back door!

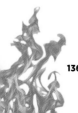

RULES FOR GOING *INSIDE* THE BUTT

- Lube. Lube. Lube! The anus doesn't naturally lubricate and the skin can tear easily with friction, so lubricant is an absolute necessity. Silicone- and water-based lubes can be used with condoms for anal sex.

- Take it slowly and proceed gradually. Begin with stimulation of the outer area only. Once you feel comfortable and relaxed, play with a small finger or toy, working your way up to larger ones as desired.

- Focus on your breathing. Relaxation is of paramount importance, and deep rhythmic breathing can help you relax your sphincter muscles and enjoy maximum pleasure.

- Accept no pain. Anal sex should not hurt! Period. It may feel a bit strange at first because you're used to using this area as a one-way, exit-only street, but differentiating between unusual sensations versus painful ones is of paramount importance. You can become more comfortable with anal pleasure if you practice tensing and relaxing the muscles in and around your anus. Experimenting with sex play that offers no penetration (with no pressure) is also a healthy way to develop comfort with this sensitive area.

- Do it yourself. And while you're at it, get to know your butt. Most people experience their first sexual arousal and orgasm from self-stimulation, because masturbation helps you become an expert in yourself. Before you dive into anal play with a partner, play with your own butt in the shower or add a lubed finger from behind while you masturbate. Learn to feel your internal and external sphincters and practice squeezing and relaxing them around your lubed finger.

- Give and receive feedback. You can't make assumptions about what your partner is feeling, so be sure to talk about what you're experiencing during penetration.

- Use toys designed specifically for the butt. If they are short toys, they should have a flared base so that they don't get sucked in and lost up there. No toy cars allowed!

- Don't cross contaminate. An object (penis, finger, toy, etc.) that has been inside the bum should not be subsequently interted into the mouth or vagina.

- Wash first. Take a sexy shower together so that you both feel clean and comfortable. Experiment with different positions to figure out the unique curves of your rectum. Practice safer sex each and every time. (See page 138.)

A FEW SEXY BUTT MOVES

Butt Massage: This should be more of a caress than a massage. Use some warming oil to draw sensual lines, ovals, circles, swirls, and figure eights all over the butt cheeks and anal opening with two fingers or warm, flat palms.

The Electric Slide: Place your lubed hand on its side as though you're performing a karate chop (but more gently) between your lover's butt cheeks near the very top. Slide it downward, curving it under toward the perineum.

Tongue Play: Slather the butt hole in your favorite flavored lube and work your tongue down the slit of the cheeks until you reach the hole. Paint sweeping ovals over it before inserting your tongue while your massage the cheeks with your hands.

Flower Power: Use well-lubed fingers to paint flower petals in a random design all around the butt hole.

Anal Beads: Visit your local sex store (or find one online) to buy your very own anal beads. Lube 'em up and have fun sliding them in and out.

Butt Worshiper: Use two hands to spread your partner's butt cheeks wide apart and dive in to eat it out with your face, nose, lips, and tongue. Suck, moan, breath, taste, and work it with all your passionate might.

Butt Master: Suck, lick, taste, and revel in the backside while your hands squeeze the butt cheeks together around your face.

Ice Cream Cone: Apply something tasty and sweet and use a wide, flat tongue to lick it off the cheeks, crack, and butt hole.

SAFER SEX

Safer sex *is* mind-blowing sex. There are some basic precautions you can take to mini-mize risk. Bear in mind that all partnered sex involves some degree of risk with regard to sexually transmitted infections (STI), so safer sex practices are a must for every sexual encounter.

Do your research and check out these sexy strategies to keep sex spicy hot.

CONDOMS

Worn over a penis, condoms come in various materials, sizes, and sexy permutations, including ribbed, nubbly, flavored, and glow-in-the-dark. Put a dollop of lube in the tip for heightened sensation and use them for manual, oral, vaginal, and anal sex to reduce the risk of STIs and unplanned pregnancy. They're so multipurpose, you can even use them for *genuphallation*—sex in which the penis is rubbed between two lubed-up knees!

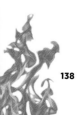

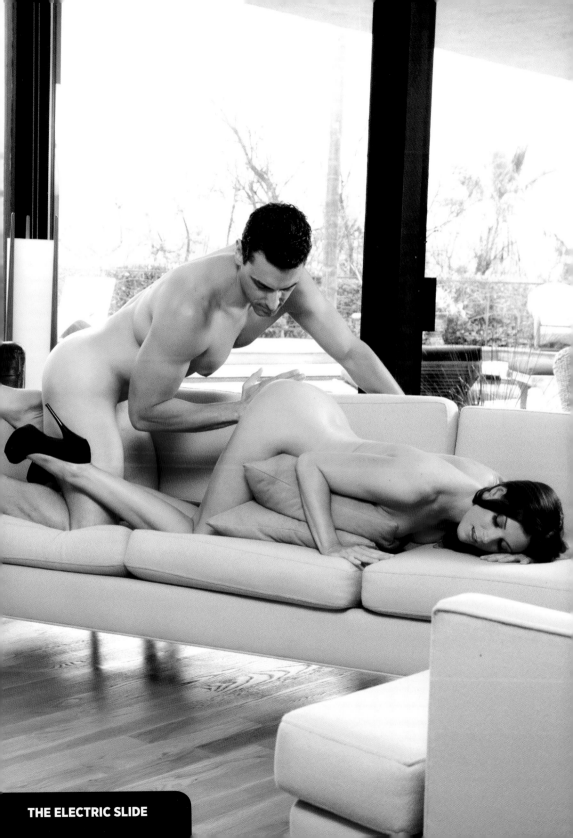

THE ELECTRIC SLIDE

FEMALE CONDOMS

Inserted into the vagina before penetrative sex, these condoms provide protection to the inner vaginal walls as well as some coverage of the vulva. A penis, toy, finger, or other object can be inserted while wearing the female condom, and it also reduces the risk of unplanned pregnancy and STIs. Removing the inner ring of the female condom is a handy alternative for penetrative anal sex that provides some additional barriers to skin contact around the anal opening.

DENTAL DAMS

These sheets of latex are placed against the vulva or anus and slathered in lube before going down and eating out. Oral sex can lead to STIs, too, so safer sex practices are a must.

GLOVES AND FINGER CONDOMS

Although manual sex (hand jobs and fingering) present lower risk for STI transmission, there is always some degree of risk. However, wearing gloves or finger condoms can offer protection and give you the peace of mind you need to keep your focus on the sex instead of worrying about unwanted consequences.

REGULAR TESTING

The most common symptom of STI infection is . . . no symptom at all! So regular testing is essential. For a list of free testing sites across North America, visit www.plannedparenthood.org/health-center.

DR. JESS SUGGESTS . . .

Cut the fingers off of a latex glove and leave the thumb on. Then cut down the opposite (non-thumb) side to create a dental dam that has an extra tube for sticking into the hold of your choice!

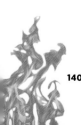

ON YOUR WAY TO MIND-BLOWING ORGASMS

BY NOW, YOU AND YOUR PARTNER ARE LIKELY WELL ON YOUR WAY to enjoying orgasms that make you weak in the knees and light in the head (unless, of course you're one of those people who skips to the *last page* of the book first!). Although you likely haven't had the chance to try out every technique yet, if you managed to at least read through the preceding chapters or even just study the pictures, you can consider yourself an expert in finger, lip, and tongue play.

Most people go through their entire lives without any formal instruction in sexual technique or pleasure, which really is unfortunate. Can you imagine learning to do anything else—like cooking, riding a bike, or playing a sport—without directions or opportunities for observation? Our finest chefs and athletes just wouldn't have developed into the superstars they are without instruction.

So give yourself a pat on the back or tell your lover to pat it for you (your back, that is), because you deserve it! Although there is always more to learn, adult sex education is probably the most exciting course of study, and you're already ahead of the game. You've taken your sexuality into your own hands and you'll be a better, more desirable lover for it. Sex is one of our greatest indulgences and there is no right way to do it, so have fun mastering new techniques and developing your own sexual style. After all, *you're* the real expert, so go ahead and start showing off your skills!

ACKNOWLEDGMENTS

Not a day goes by that I don't count my blessings, as I am surrounded by wonderful people.

Thank you to my friends and family for putting up with a daughter, sister, and friend whose professional title alone makes people blush, squirm and whisper. I can't promise it will get any easier, but at least blushing looks good on you—especially you, Mom.

I also owe much appreciation to all those who have generously supported my academic and professional development over the years. Special thanks to June Larkin, Stefanie Lopacinski-Welch, Jan Haskings-Winner, and Daven Seebarran: your support has been invaluable. And to Wendy Miller, Emily Sinclair and the rest of the *SWING* crew: thanks for putting up with my manuscript writing on-set and for providing visual inspiration aplenty.

Much appreciation and credit goes to the team at Quiver Books who made the writing, editing and publishing process painless (for me, at least). A huge thank you to Kevin Mulroy, Holly Randall, Robert Brandt, Meg Sniegoski, Karen Levy, Leah Jenness, and Traffic Design Consultants. Extra special thanks to Jill Alexander and John Gettings, whose patience and kind words during the editing process kept me motivated and focused.

Finally, a lifetime of appreciation goes to my partner and biggest fan, Brandon Ware. You offer inspiration, love, and support to no end. Thanks for forcing me to celebrate the small stuff and for inspiring me to dream big.

xoxo

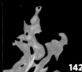

ABOUT THE AUTHOR

JESSICA O'REILLY (Dr. Jess) is a sexologist, relationship expert and television personality who travels the globe to promote healthy and deliciously pleasurable sex. From hosting PlayboyTV's top-rated reality show, SWING, to running beachside couples' retreats in the Caribbean, she relishes in every moment.

With a Ph.D. in human sexuality and an extensive resume of international experience, Dr. Jess has become the go-to expert for all things sexual. Her speaking engagements at clinical conferences, colleges/universities, corporate retreats, and entertainment events draw sold-out crowds and she keeps audiences coming back for more with her intimate knowledge of S-E-X, warm personality, and healthy sense of humor.

Dr. Jess has worked with over 1,200 couples from all corners of the world to improve communication, enhance trust, overcome sexual challenges, and keep the sexual flame burning in long-term relationships. She also offers sexuality education and support for special needs youth, HIV–positive clientele, classroom teachers, cancer survivors, parents, teens, and clinicians.

To learn more about Dr. Jess, please visit her website at www.SexWithDrJess.com